MANAGED BEHAVIORAL HEALTH CARE

MANAGED BEHAVIORAL HEALTH CARE

An Industry Perspective

Edited by

SHARON A. SHUEMAN, PH.D.

Principal, Shueman Troy & Associates
Pasadena, California

WARWICK G. TROY, PH.D., M.P.H.

Director of Research
California School of Professional Psychology
Los Angeles
Principal, Shueman Troy & Associates
Pasadena, California

and

SAMUEL L. MAYHUGH, PH.D.

President, Integrated Behavioral Health
Laguna Hills, California

With a Foreword by
Peter Boland, Ph.D.

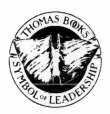

CHARLES C THOMAS • PUBLISHER
Springfield • Illinois • U.S.A.

Published and Distributed Throughout the World by

CHARLES C THOMAS • PUBLISHER
2600 South First Street
Springfield, Illinois 62794-9265

© *1994 by* CHARLES C THOMAS • PUBLISHER

ISBN 0-398-05897-0

Library of Congress Catalog Card Number: 93-34578

With THOMAS BOOKS *careful attention is given to all details of manufacturing
and design. It is the Publisher's desire to present books that are satisfactory as to
their physical qualities and artistic possibilities and appropriate for their particular
use.* THOMAS BOOKS *will be true to those laws of quality that assure a good
name and good will.*

Printed in the United States of America
SC-R-3

Library of Congress Cataloging-in-Publication Data

Managed behavioral health care : an industry perspective / edited by
Sharon A. Shueman, Warwick G. Troy, and Samuel L. Mayhugh; with
foreword by Peter Boland.
    p.   cm.
  Includes bibliographical references and index.
  ISBN 0-398-05897-0
  1. Managed care plans (Medical care)—United States. 2. Mental
health services—United States. 3. Psychiatry—Practice—United
States. I. Shueman, Sharon A. II. Troy, Warwick G. III. Mayhugh,
Samuel L.
  [DNLM: 1. Mental Health Services—organization & administration—
United States. 2. Personal Health Services—organization &
administration—United States. 3. Managed Care Programs—
organization & administration—United States. WM 30 M2652 1994]
RA790.5.M287   1994
362.2'068—dc20
DNLM/DLC
for Library of Congress   93-34578
                                            CIP

CONTRIBUTORS

DONALD F. ANDERSON, PH.D.
Leader, National Mental Health Practice
National Medical Audit Inc.
A unit of William M. Mercer Inc.
San Francisco, California

JEFFREY L. BERLANT, M.D., PH.D.
Senior Consultant Mental Health and Substance Abuse
National Medical Audit Inc.
A unit of William M. Mercer Inc.
San Francisco, California

PETER BOLAND, PH.D.
President, Boland Healthcare Inc.
Berkeley, California

ELIZABETH Q. BULATAO, M.A.
Communications Development Officer
American Psychological Association
Washington, D.C.

NICHOLAS A. CUMMINGS, PH.D., LITT.D.
President
Foundation for Behavioral Health
Founding Chairman and CEO (Retired)
American Biodyne Inc.
South San Francisco, California

PATRICK H. DeLEON, PH.D., J.D., M.P.H.
Administrative Assistant
Senator Daniel Inouye, U.S. Senate
Washington, D.C.

HERBERT DÖRKEN, PH.D.
Registered Lobbyist, California
Scientific Director
Foundation for Behavioral Health
South San Francisco, California

MARY G. HENDERSON, Ph.D.
Consultant
Hewitt Associates
Lincolnshire, Illinois

NANCY E. LANE, Ph.D.
Clinical Director APM East
American PsychManagement
Arlington, Virginia

BRIAN L. MAYHUGH, Ph.D.
Director of Clinical Services
Integrated Behavioral Health
Laguna Hills, California

SAMUEL L. MAYHUGH, Ph.D.
President and CEO
Integrated Behavioral Health
Laguna Hills, California

ARNOLD MILSTEIN, M.D., M.P.H.
President, National Medical Audit Inc.
A unit of William M. Mercer Inc.
Associate Clinical Professor
University of California San Francisco
San Francisco, California

MICHAEL S. PALLAK, Ph.D.
Executive Vice President and Vice President for Research
Foundation for Behavioral Health
South San Francisco, California

NORMAN R. PENNER, M.P.H.
Assistant Vice President and Executive Director
Ethix Behavioral Services
Beaverton, Oregon

BETTIE REINHARDT, R.N., M.P.H.
Director of Operations
National Psych Reviews
San Diego, California

CHARLES L. ROGERSON, Ph.D.
Director of Healthcare Data Modeling
TDS Healthcare Systems Corporation
San Jose, California

GARY L. SHEPHERD, M.D. (Deceased)
Vice President, Medical Services
National Psych Reviews
San Diego, California

SHARON A. SHUEMAN, Ph.D.
Principal
Shueman Troy & Associates
Pasadena, California

WARWICK G. TROY, Ph.D., M.P.H.
Director of Research
California School of Professional Psychology, Los Angeles
Principal
Shueman Troy & Associates
Pasadena, California

GARY R. VandenBos, Ph.D.
Executive Director
Publications and Communications
American Psychological Association
Washington, D.C.

This book is dedicated to the memory of
Gary L. Shepherd
and
Harl H. Young

FOREWORD

The behavioral health field is at a critical crossroad. Care givers must decide if they want to actively shape policies that will affect their patients, practice, and institutions, or passively accept the current business-oriented requirements of managed health care.

Behavioral health professionals no longer have a choice about whether to participate in managed care. It is the dominant force in the health care industry. The only realistic decision for psychiatrists, psychologists, psychiatric nurses, social workers, counselors, and psychiatric treatment facilities involves the particular forms participation will take.

There are important lessons to be learned from the experience of medical-surgical service providers in adapting to managed care. During the 1980s, most providers failed to give purchasers and payers adequate documentation about *how* their health care dollars were spent, *why* they were used in that manner, *what* alternative treatment options were available, or *what* was achieved by way of treatment outcomes or patient functioning. As a result, the customer lost faith in the supplier's ability to provide high quality mental health and substance abuse services at acceptable prices. Employers and payers responded with burdensome cost containment mechanisms and administrative controls. These include benefit restrictions, utilization review procedures, quality assurance mechanisms, and tighter reimbursement formulas based on diagnostic related groups (DRGs) and volume discounts.

Behavioral health providers were spared these restrictions and impositions for a time, but this is no longer the case. They failed to learn the lessons provided by medical-surgical care and they now face the problem of winning back the trust of powerful "distribution channels" (i.e., insurers, delivery systems, managed behavioral health organizations and government), benefit designers, and policy makers now controlling the flow of mental health services.

The managed care industry does not have answers to many difficult behavioral health care issues. These include balancing patient need with appropriate cost management, improving long-term quality within the context of one-year contracts, and documenting performance with few agreed-upon standards of care or methods of measuring treatment outcomes. The problems inherent in funding and rendering appropriate care for chronic conditions, especially to medically under served groups, is a particularly vexing issue. Answers to such questions must be sought through greater collaboration and cooperation between behavioral health professionals and managed care delivery systems.

In a managed care environment, successful behavioral health practitioners are those who adapt or change their practice styles to embrace (among other techniques) the short-term, outpatient-focused interventions favored by managed care organizations. For many clinicians, this orientation will require retraining and acquiring new skills.

Practice guidelines will play an increasingly important role in determining the right mix of mental health services and care settings. Thus, behavioral health servicing will evolve from treatment delivered according to local community standards to treatment based on protocols reflecting scientific findings about likely outcomes. Clinical efficacy (as determined by rigorous research) and cost-effectiveness will become the central element of the framework for directing managed mental health care companies and managed care delivery systems.

Collaboration between care givers and structural integration among different professional disciplines are replacing adversarial relationships and fragmented care. One of the clearest trends in managed care—and one to which behavioral health care providers must adapt—is the emergence of integrated clinical networks which emphasize primary care. When such networks are equipped with integrated, computerized information systems, more effective and efficient coordination of medical and behavioral health services can be achieved. Different types of practitioners and practice protocols can be brought together and managed. And, if medical offset factors are taken seriously by managed care companies, behavioral health care may become a mainstay of primary care referral.

The integration of behavioral health with primary medical care can result in better service quality and better cost management. Many individuals with psychiatric disorders seek care through primary health care systems. When "gatekeeper" approaches in such systems are properly integrated with behavioral health, timely referrals to mental health professionals can be made. The medical offset effect results in reducing overall cost and improving quality of care when appropriate referral and service coordination occur. Gatekeeper models do not necessarily reduce costs or improve quality, however. Administrative hurdles and inadequate clinical judgment by gatekeepers can create barriers to needed care.

Electronic linkage among providers, monitoring organizations, and payers has the potential to bring together outcome evaluation, practice management, and reimbursement. When payers are able to accurately document costs and results, they will be able to link compensation to the actual performance of the delivery system.

Cost management and quality improvement are inextricably linked when the overall goal is improving health status and level of functioning. Behavioral health professionals must work collaboratively with other health professionals in the managed care industry to determine how to best integrate behavioral and medical-surgical services for individual beneficiaries and specific population groups. This requires providers to adopt the role of team member rather than independent practitioner. It also requires them to ask tough questions on behalf of the patient *and* the payer about the appropriateness and effectiveness of different treatments and settings and their relative contributions to improving continuity and quality of care. Under managed care, professional autonomy will give way to an interdisciplinary approach to managing patient services guided by empirically-based standards of efficacy. In short, accountability to patients and payers will become the hallmark of managed behavioral health care in the 1990s.

Managed care can be seen by behavioral health practitioners as a dangerous threat or as a new opportunity to influence how care is provided as part of an integrated financing and service system. Now is the time for behavioral health professionals to clarify their vision of how to improve the quality of services, coverage, and accountability.

Health care reform initiatives at the state and national levels are struggling with how to redefine the role and *value* of mental health services in society. It is critical for behavioral health service providers to assume a primary role in this activity and in determining how to provide needed care within new budget constraints. This is the foremost challenge facing the profession today.

Managed Behavioral Health Care thoughtfully examines the market forces propelling behavioral health care practitioners into managed behavioral health care systems, as well as the social and cultural forces inhibiting change. It provides a balanced assessment of the strengths and weaknesses of current managed care systems and offers the insight of managed care experts, many of whom have been involved in the industry since its inception. Finally, it suggests what the professions must do to survive—and preserve the treatment values upon which they were founded.

This book constitutes a valuable contribution to the literature on managed care and will be of great interest to a wide range of readers, including behavioral health professionals, students preparing to enter these professions, policy makers, and those involved in the development and implementation of these new managed care delivery systems.

PETER BOLAND, PH.D.
President
Boland Healthcare Inc.
Berkeley, California
Editor
Managed Care Quarterly

PREFACE

This book is about a relatively new industry, behavioral health services provided under managed systems: *managed behavioral health
care*. Behavioral health embraces the traditional areas of mental health
and chemical dependency but includes, in addition, the many applications of the behavioral sciences which have been shown to affect the
physical as well as the behavioral and emotional aspects of human
functioning. Behavioral health services would, for example, include
treatment for chronic pain, counseling to assist in recovery from illness
or surgery, and employee assistance counseling to deal with problems
affecting work performance. It encompasses the fields of behavioral
medicine and health psychology.

Not surprisingly, since it is in a formative stage of development,
managed behavioral health care as an industry is characterized by significant variation in the organization, procedures, and products of its services management systems. While variation is generally held to be the
enemy of quality, it is also the inevitable companion of innovation—
particularly on a large scale.

This variation in managed care is reflected in the approaches to the
topics taken by the authors of the chapters in this book. The reader will,
for example, be exposed to different perceptions of the case management
process and contrasting views on quality assurance and accountability
mechanisms. This is to be expected. None of the authors was exposed to
managed care issues in his or her professional training programs and,
until only very recently, the literature on managed care has been practically non-existent. What these authors know and believe about managed
care is very largely a function of their personal experiences as clinicians
providing services in managed systems, as program developers creating
them, as program administrators directing them, and as external evaluators
making judgments about them. Although most of the authors share a
background in clinical applications, their professional preparation has

been in diverse areas (e.g., psychiatry, psychiatric nursing, clinical psychology, public health), each of which provides a unique orientation to health services delivery.

One of the inescapable consequences of an innovation such as managed behavioral health care is controversy. A person with even a casual interest in health care can not be unaware of the criticisms of managed care coming from provider and, to a lesser extent, consumer and employer communities. The typical criticisms are that managed systems focus on cost containment at the expense of quality and that they are inflexible and inhospitable to provider and beneficiary alike. That quality concerns are now paramount is perhaps ironic in view of the fact that, in the context of the uncontrolled service delivery mechanisms which preceded managed care, few people worried about quality. Quality assurance was seen as a regulatory responsibility, something imposed on service providers from the outside. Certainly, issues relating to process and outcome assessment and quality management were not, nor have ever been, included in the professional training curricula of the various disciplines.

Managed care in its current forms does not constitute a panacea for the myriad cost and quality problems attendant on health services provision. The attempts to solve problems in the industry have, in many instances, created new ones, and managed care has raised more questions about cost and quality issues than it has answered. On the other hand, its positive contributions to date have been to raise awareness about the need for accountability in health services and to impose some structure on the previously unstructured world of independent practice. Managed care has created service *systems,* however imperfect. Having a system does not guarantee that quality of services will be assured or their costs contained. It does, however, provide an essential foundation for addressing these issues.

As the title of this book suggests, it is about an industry largely from the perspective of those within the industry. It is to be hoped that the potential lack of perspective inherent in such an approach is minimized by the significant variation in the disciplinary background of the contributors, their individual roles, experiences, and professional values stances. The problematic nature of the industry is sufficient for an apologist approach to be considered as much an impertinence as a lapse in professional judgment. Nonetheless, the thesis of this book and its motive force is that in the rapidly changing, essentially chaotic world of managed behavioral health care are many of the crucial elements of a large-scale social experiment—however haphazardly contrived—and that there is an obligation to analyze phenomena discerned in this laboratory from the point of view of the participant observer.

There is a long tradition of well-conducted health services research within the large prepaid plans, the HMOs. The managed behavioral health care industry rather desperately needs the attention of such applied scholarly endeavours. Indeed, a small number of managed behavioral health care companies have initiated promising services utilization and outcomes-based research programs; such approaches are, however, the exception.

The models presented and discussed throughout this book relate primarily to private sector, employer-funded managed care programs—the sector with which the authors are most familiar and in which most managed behavioral health services have been delivered. The lack of attention to public sector care in no way reflects the editors' estimation of its importance vis-à-vis managed care. Clearly, managed models have significant potential for publicly funded services. And there can be no question that a more effective integration of public and private sector programs is a necessary prerequisite to improving the capacity of privately funded programs to deal with issues of chronicity: something that they currently do relatively poorly. The prevailing attitude is that problems of chronic, disabling mental illness are more appropriately dealt with by public sector programs. Indeed, Schlesinger and Mechanic[1] have suggested that the challenges may be most usefully addressed by specialist managed care entities such as social health maintenance organizations (SHMO). Regardless of the form of the arrangements which emerge over the next decade, or whether public-private partnerships develop to deal with the problems of the severely and chronically mentally ill, the role of services management will no doubt be an important one. The current discourse on managed competition prompted by the Health Reform Task Force would seem to ensure this.

It is hoped that this book can provide a better sense of what goes on in the industry, what seems to work, and what might be fixed. The editors

---

1. Schlesinger, M. & Mechanic, D. (1993). Challenges for managed competition from chronic illness. *Health Affairs*, Supplement, 123–137.

are not only buoyed by a prevailing sense of optimism, but also impressed by the industry's signal achievements, accomplishments largely obscured by the contentiousness of the debate which so characterizes the field.

Sharon A. Shueman
Warwick G. Troy
Samuel L. Mayhugh

ACKNOWLEDGMENTS

The editors would like to acknowledge four people whose work has greatly influenced our thinking on issues of quality and accountability in health services. These people are Russell L. Bent, Robert H. Brook, Nicholas A. Cummings, and Avedis Donabedian.

We would also like to thank Brian S. Gould for his support and significant contributions during the early days of the development of this book.

CONTENTS

MANAGED BEHAVIORAL HEALTH CARE

PART I
THE MOVE TOWARD ACCOUNTABILITY

PART I: INTRODUCTORY NOTE

Chapters 1 and 2 provide background for the movement toward accountability in behavioral health services which began in the late 1970s. Prior to managed care, mental health and chemical dependency services were provided without any effective controls on cost or quality. Providers delivered services according to their own style and preference, and payers paid the bill, generally without question. While, in theory, the provider was accountable to the patient, the inequalities in knowledge and power within the therapeutic relationship meant that patients were rarely in a position to assert their rights as consumers.

In Chapter 1, Shueman, Troy, and Mayhugh set a context for the changes which were to come by describing the health care financing structure of the 1970s and the ways in which it not only provided few mechanisms for dealing with problems in service delivery, but also exacerbated those problems. They discuss also other critical variables, most notably the mental health professional training programs and professional socialization process, which contributed to an environment in which accountability was devalued.

The tide began to turn in the late 1970s when the federal government instituted external regulatory mechanisms intended to make mental health and chemical dependency service providers more responsive to the needs of payers and consumers. In Chapter 2, Penner describes these pioneering initiatives within the Civilian Health and Medical Program of the Uniformed Services (CHAMPUS) which were intended specifically to deal with spiralling health care costs and reports of serious patient abuse in some sectors of the service system. To increase acceptance of their efforts within the professional communities, the federal government sought the assistance of the two major mental health professional associations—the American Psychiatric Association and the American Psychological Association—to develop the system for monitoring services. It was, in some ways, a naive attempt, but one which established a vital precedent: that service providers had an obligation to respond to efforts by purchasers attempting to make *informed* determinations of necessity and appropriateness of services they were buying.

The guild-oriented nature of the professional associations made it impossible for them to sustain their accountability efforts, but by the time the two associations acceded to member opposition and gave up these activities a number of similar review programs had been established within the private sector. The bold experiment by the government had evolved into a myriad of entrepreneurial models, each of which had its own strengths and weaknesses and each of which contributed something to the development of the managed care industry. Again, in Chapter 1, Shueman, Troy, and Mayhugh provide a typical example of a modern managed care program and discuss some of the major issues which challenge the continued development of managed behavioral health care.

Chapter 1

PRINCIPLES AND ISSUES IN
MANAGED BEHAVIORAL HEALTH CARE

Sharon A. Shueman, Warwick G. Troy, and Samuel L. Mayhugh

This chapter is focused on the basic principles and key issues within managed behavioral health care as it is currently practiced in the U.S. It includes a discussion of the health services and financing environment which existed prior to the early 1980s and which created the need and provided the foundation for managed care. Also highlighted are some of the specific cost and quality concerns which prompted organizations to begin to develop a range of innovative strategies to better manage the behavioral health service system. A typical example of a managed care program is provided to clarify how the fundamental dimensions of managed care are manifest in formal arrangements between purchasers and services management organizations. The chapter concludes with a brief discussion of the issues and controversies which surround the managed care industry.

THE ENVIRONMENT THAT ENGENDERED MANAGED CARE

One of the most serious problems affecting the health status of Americans is the weak association between need for health care, on the one hand, and accessibility to such care, on the other. Historically, market forces together with life circumstances have functionally determined who has access to needed services. Persons whose access to services is mediated by their qualifying for state and federal entitlement programs or public care are often severely restricted in the types and amount of behavioral health care available to them. Those without employer-sponsored benefit plans and who do not qualify for any of the public programs are even more restricted in access. Persons whose health plan provides coverage for behavioral health care generally do have access to a range of such services. Among these people, however, problems of over servicing as well as inappropriate servicing are likely to be at least as serious as under servicing. Much of behavioral health care has been directed neither at people with a significant disability nor at those who are severely at risk.

In the U.S., the lack of a developed role for centralized planning in the health system, the dominance of market forces, and the absence of a single payer system all act against the evolution of a rational relationship between need and access to service. Given the relative absence of macro restraints available in many other countries (e.g., universal coverage combined with some system of cost management such as global budgeting), the malaise that afflicts the U.S. health system will certainly continue.

It is conceivable, of course, that the recent apparent movement toward a national health system could in time result in significant improvements in health care financing and organization in the U.S. If so, managed care in general, and managed behavioral health care in particular, could be effectively poised for a significantly enhanced role in what could at last become a *system* of health care in America. In the current environment, however, if health status is not inevitably to decline, it must increasingly fall to micro approaches to deal with some of the burden, a burden exacerbated by catastrophic budget shortfalls in public sector care, and reduced availability of corporate funds for benefit support in the private sector.

The incorporation of innovations at the level of health services production is essential to confronting these seemingly overwhelming challenges. At the same time, the industry must contend with the historical antipathy of the provider community toward fiscal and service accountability. It is in this context that the potential of the financing and service arrangements, known in all their variations as "managed care," must be acknowledged.

In attempting to identify the unique promise of managed care, it is less important to distinguish among its many variants than to understand the fundamental principles of the models. The majority of managed care arrangements share the following basic principles:

- Providers and clients are integral components of a larger functionally integrated system.
- Providers, and the larger systems of which they are a part, are held professionally accountable for their services and often assume some financial "risk."

- These integrated systems directly accept responsibility for client outcomes.

The potential contributions of managed care systems in provision of behavioral health services may exceed those which are possible in general medical-surgical care given the historically low baseline of quality in the former. This is not to say that the latter types of services have been free of cost and quality problems. It is to say that the problems of behavioral health services (to date, defined mainly as mental health and chemical dependency treatment) have been more pervasive and more serious. This is due to a number of factors, including:

- The lack of application of appropriate scientific techniques to questions of efficacy of behavioral health services;
- The proliferation of providers (psychiatrists, psychologists, social workers, marriage and family therapists, psychiatric nurses, mental health counselors, chemical dependency counselors, EAP counselors) who, as a group, do not share common standards of education, training, or professional development;
- Graduate training programs which, by and large, have imbued providers with a lack of appreciation for, and sometimes even a distinctly negative attitude about, the necessity for accountability to a larger system;
- Lack of a common approach to treatment between, as well as within, provider (professional discipline) groups, related either to the dominance of theoretical orientation or the lack of adequate training;
- Lack of expertise about mental health and chemical dependency problems and services within the payer community which prevented it from asking legitimate questions about the necessity and appropriateness of provider-endorsed services.

This is a powerful and disturbingly negative legacy, and it suggests that the challenges confronting the managed care companies extend far beyond the level of the individual episode of care. The challenges also relate directly to the system of education, training, and professional socialization of providers; the discriminatory attitude toward (and consequent lack of knowledge about) mental health which exists within the health system; and the absence of any effective mechanism for bringing research and evaluation techniques to bear on behavioral health service delivery (VandenBos, 1993).

Factors Influencing the Development of Managed Care

Obviously, cost has been a significant motivator in the development of managed care. The following terse litany from Englund and Vaccaro (1991), for example, conveys the severity of the problem for corporate purchasers of health and mental health services.

> In 1990, employer/purchasers saw another 21% increase in their health care expenditures, despite cost containment efforts spanning more than a decade. Mental health and chemical dependency services [have]... cost increases of up to 60% per year.... Employers report that mental and substance abuse disorders are among the most frequent short-term disability cases. Both the number and duration of these cases are on the rise, driving up the expense of both disability and health insurance (p. 129).

Previous Attempts to Manage Costs

Prior to managed care (excluding certain HMOs), attempts to manage mental health costs tended to favor *ad hoc* approaches such as defining a limited benefit. Typical benefit plans provided for a fixed amount (e.g., $2,000) to be reimbursed per year, limited the amount reimbursed per procedure (e.g., 50% of the "usual and customary fee" to a maximum of $40 per therapy session), or limited the quantity of services paid for (e.g., 20 therapy sessions and 30 days of hospitalization per year). At the same time, cost-effective alternatives such as day treatment and outpatient drug rehabilitation programs were generally not included in the benefit plan, since insurance companies believed they would only add to the total cost of services. Finally, benefit plans used diagnosis rather than services as a basis for reimbursement (Goldman, Adler, Berlant et al., 1993). This resulted in, among other things, inaccurate reporting of diagnoses by providers and a consequent diminution of the quality of the data supporting decision making in the payment system.

As a result of poorly conceived benefit structures, people who needed particular amounts or types of services often could not afford them, while high cost inpatient services were often used unnecessarily. In short, the large proportion of patients whose needs were not consistent with the benefit structure received inappropriate care, or no care. Benefit arrangements lacked the flexibility which would allow care to be tailored to the unique needs of individual patients. Even when utilization review was conducted, it was generally done retrospectively, after treatment was completed, at which time any denial was very likely to result in significant financial hardship to the patient. Sadly, system flexibility was limited to the ingenuity of service providers as they sought to exploit the benefit system "in the interest of the patient."

Problems in the Service System

While highly significant, costs were by no means the only factor motivating payers to find ways to gain more control of services. Mental health and chemical dependency services presented consumers and purchasers with several other problems, the scope and severity of which were largely unmatched in general health care. The very early attempts at managing behavioral health care took place partially in response to what stakeholders perceived as an unpredictable and essentially chaotic service system. The lack of predictability and general confusion were grounded in the stakeholders' severely restricted understanding of services and service providers, together with great (and to many observers, unacceptable) variation in the level of quality.

CONFUSION ABOUT TREATMENT OPTIONS. Purchasers—usually insurance companies—were confused by the provider-sanctioned definitions and treatment alternatives for mental and emotional problems. This confusion was partly due to the fact that the third parties often had minimal access to knowledgable staff or rational resources expert in mental health care. It was heightened, however, by what the purchasers saw within the service system. For example, they were forced to contend with provider sanctioning of apparently well-functioning individuals receiving intensive outpatient therapy over long periods of time; with patients with the same diagnosis being treated in dramatically different ways—often dependent on the idiosyncratic theoretical orientation of the providers; and with treatment approaches seemingly related to nothing more than services covered in the benefit. Passive and unempowered purchasers also had to accept provider groups whose training programs and approaches differed markedly from one another, but who treated the same types of patients and problems using the same techniques.

QUALITY CONCERNS. The second factor which contributed to the chaos which seemed to purchasers to typify mental health and chemical dependency services was an apparent inability or unwillingness of many service providers to consistently adhere to the accepted tenets of professionalism and quality in service delivery. What appeared to pervade the system was an unacceptably low level of quality together with patterns of practice oriented toward leveraging maximal gains from third party payers (e.g., providing unnecessary services or providing service in unnecessarily high intensity settings).

Increasingly, payers came to view providers as groups unable to identify unambiguously what they were trying to achieve in treatment and derisive of those who suggested that they should focus on the improvement of functioning at the expense of changing the patient's underlying character structure. Too often improvement, if it came, seemed too modest to the increasingly cynical payer community to justify the significant investment in time and money made in treatment. Such negative attitudes were seen to be supported by the periodic reports in the popular press about instances of unprofessional or unethical behavior or incompetence on the part of service providers resulting in abuse and, sometimes, injury to patients (Asher, 1981).

Needed System Reform

From the perspective of the payer, then, the prevailing mental health and chemical dependency service system came to be seen as untenable. Even if essentially *ad hoc* benefit related cost-control mechanisms had been successful in limiting the costs of mental health and chemical dependency services, the very real issues of necessity, appropriateness, and quality would have remained. There was virtually nothing in the financing system to guarantee that money spent was appropriately spent, or that money saved was appropriately saved. This was a particularly critical issue for those employers who believed that the problems among employees resulting from the lack of appropriate and effective mental health and chemical dependency treatment would result in added costs to the company (e.g., in terms of reduced productivity; increased sick leave, turnover, and injuries on the job; and increased use of medical services).

Crucial system reform of existing benefit and financing strategies would provide not only for flexibility at the point of service, but also for effective mechanisms for monitoring necessity, appropriateness, and quality of care. The objectives, then, of such a system would be to:

- ensure access to necessary services;
- manage costs;
- assure adequate quality; and
- significantly enhance the probability of successful clinical outcomes.

The Beginnings of System Reform

Insurance companies were not among the first organizations to attempt to deal with the cost and quality problems in behavioral health services. One of the reasons for this was because of a lack of knowledge and expertise within these organizations. Another reason was probably related to the functional independence of payer and provider as embedded in law and regulation. Only if a payer organization functioned as a prepaid health plan could it become involved "in the business" of health services (Vaughan, 1986).

A third and more pragmatic reason was that mental health services costs, historically, were relatively insignificant. In comparison with medical-surgical services, mental health and chemical dependency were a relatively small part (often only 5–10%) of the health care budget for any payer. Moreover, insurance policies were generally "experience rated". This meant that if costs for behavioral health services increased, the insurance company would renegotiate the contract during the next contracting cycle and, based on the utilization experience of the employee group, raise the premiums. Payers were generally not financially at risk for longer than a defined financial cycle, so it really mattered little to them in the longer term whether or not costs increased.

Rather than originating with insurance companies, then, the first significant attempts at solutions to the cost and quality problems in mental health came from the two major mental health professional associations, the American Psychiatric Association and the American Psychological Association, in the guise of the federally supported CHAMPUS review programs (Shueman & Penner, 1988). Subsequent initiatives originated with specialty review organizations developed and managed primarily by mental health professionals who were responding to a market created by the growing number of self-insured employers. Insurance companies did enter this arena, but relatively late, often by buying existing review or managed care organizations.

WHAT CHARACTERIZES MANAGED CARE?

The development of the managed care industry has seen an increase in the size and complexity of both corporate entities and service delivery models. The models exist as various structures, including the health maintenance organization (HMO), preferred provider organization (PPO), exclusive provider organization (EPO), the independent practice association (IPA), and the point-of-service plan (POS). Within each of these models are a multitude of variations in both structure and function of management, financing, and service delivery. Common to all models, however, are four key dimensions on which these variations occur. The dimensions are:

- *Selective contracting* in which providers and managed care companies agree on a set of business "ground rules" under which the providers will work and the managed care company will pay them. Generally, such arrangements are either *preferred* (providers outside of the network may be reimbursed for services) or *exclusive* (only network providers may be reimbursed).

- *A process for assessing and managing services* based on a system of utilization review or case management; explicit objectives are to *facilitate access* to necessary and appropriate care and *ensure the adequacy and cost-effectiveness* of services provided.

- *A financing structure,* typically stipulating that the case management organization will assume some amount of financial risk under a capitated system (Koch, 1988) and services will be reimbursed under a fee system negotiated by the company and providers. Increasingly, providers are also being asked to assume some financial risk.

- *A benefit design* which defines covered services and includes financial and other incentives for providers and patients to encourage early intervention, use of contracted providers, and use of lower intensity (more cost-effective) services.

These four dimensions and their interdependencies are more easily understood in context of an example.

An Example of a Managed Care Partnership

The XYZ Company is a large (15,000 employees in 12 states nationwide) corporation which has contracted with ABC Behavioral Health Services, Inc. to manage all mental health and chemical dependency benefits and services to its employees and their dependents. The managed care arrangement has the following characteristics.

Selective Contracting

ABC is a specialty managed behavioral health care company which contracts in 23 states with preferred individual and institutional providers who have agreed to cooperate with the case management personnel and review process and to accept the fees offered by ABC in return for referrals. In the case of individual providers this is a set fee per 45–50 minute session of $90 for psychiatrists, $90 for (doctoral level) psychologists, $70 for clinical social workers, and $60 for other licensed masters level professionals. For many providers the fees are a discount from their typical charge, but for others they are not. For a few, the fees are actually above their usual and customary. ABC has attempted to maintain a network which is large enough to provide easy and timely access for prospective patients, but small enough to ensure a relatively high number of referrals for each provider.

In the case of institutional providers such as acute care hospitals, residential treatment centers, structured outpatient or day treatment programs, and home-based programs for mental illness and chemical dependency. ABC's provider relations director has negotiated a separate fee with each organization (in essence, trying to get the "best deal" for ABC that she can get). For inpatient and residential services, fees are on a per diem basis, with the per diem covering all services specified in the contract (usually all but daily visits by an "attending" professional). For structured outpatient programs, such as chemical dependency rehabilitation, the fee covers the entire course of treatment. While these fees are individually negotiated with each organization or program, in all cases they are significantly lower than would typically be charged to a self-paying patient or to a patient covered by a traditional insurance plan.

The system designed for XYZ is a "preferred" rather than "exclusive" provider organization. This means that patients may, under some circumstances, receive reimbursement for services provided by non-network individuals or institutions, but certain provisions of the benefit are designed to discourage this (see below).

A Process for Managing Services

All beneficiaries are given a toll free phone number which they may call to obtain a referral to a network professional or institutional provider. In response to a call and assisted by a computer-based set of protocols and guidelines, a case manager employed by ABC makes a preliminary assessment of need and determines the type of provider and treatment setting most likely to be appropriate for the patient. For example, if there is evidence the patient may need medication, a referral is made to a psychiatrist. The case manager gives the caller the name of a provider close to the patient's home and calls the provider to notify him or her of the referral. The case manager may even schedule an initial appointment for the caller. Referrals may also occur through the company's employee assistance program (EAP) to ABC or directly to a provider in ABC's network.

REPORTING REQUIREMENTS. Outpatient providers must submit to ABC's case managers a problem-oriented (Bent, 1988) written treatment plan for all patients whom they intend to see for more than three sessions. The plan must describe problems and state goals in functional terms, it must describe clear strategies whereby these goals will be achieved, and it must provide an expected time frame for completion of treatment. Reimbursement for more than three outpatient sessions depends upon review and approval by a case manager of such a plan. The case manager has the option of approving payment for the plan as presented, approving it contingent on specific changes, approving a smaller number of sessions than requested and reviewing the case after that number of sessions has elapsed, or disapproving payment for the services as described in the plan.

For services delivered by institutional providers, such as acute inpatient, inpatient rehabilitation for chemical dependency, residential treatment, home-based programs, day treatment, and structured outpatient programs, services must be approved by a case manager before the patient is admitted or, in the case of a genuine emergency, within 24 hours after admission. The facility or program obtains pre-authorization by calling the toll free number. For services which are approved, the case manager requests periodic progress reviews in the form of proposed continued treatment plans, again expressed in a problem-oriented format, on which he or she bases decisions about continued reimbursement for the services.

SERVICE MONITORING. During the course of treatment, ABC's case managers have the option of discussing with providers anything which they believe may be relevant to the necessity or appropriateness of care. Providers are also encouraged to contact case managers if they believe the resources or support of the case manager could be helpful. This could occur, for example, with a non-compliant patient or a patient who may have atypical service needs. To help increase consistency in decision-making across case managers and raise the level of quality of services, ABC maintains a set of research-based practice guidelines which set out diagnosis-specific treatment strategies that have been shown in empirical studies to be effective. Case managers use these as general guides when reviewing treatment plans (e.g., if a treatment plan differs markedly from the guidelines the case manager may question the appropriateness of the plan). Final decisions about reimbursement are always based on the clinical judgment of case managers or consultant (peer) reviewers.

At the end of treatment, providers submit a written discharge summary which includes their estimate of the patient's prognosis, and case managers conduct mail or phone follow-up with all patients. Six months after treatment has terminated patients are surveyed regarding the adequacy of their current functioning and are asked to evaluate the clinical and administrative services they received.

Financing Structure

XYZ is a "self-insured" company with regard to its employees' mental health and chemical dependency treatment needs. This means that rather than buy a traditional indemnity policy from an insurance company and allow that company to take the financial risk (or possibly realize a financial benefit if utilization turns out to be low), XYZ purchases the administrative and clinical services directly from ABC company. Such an arrangement allows XYZ to save money on certain overhead and premium fees imposed by insurance companies, to have more of a direct influence on the structure of the service delivery system, and to more closely monitor certain aspects of services. ABC reviews and pays claims submitted by the providers, and funds are transferred as needed from XYZ to its claim account which is administered by ABC. ABC has agreed to manage all necessary mental health and chemical dependency services required by XYZ's employees and dependents and to pay claims for a monthly fee of $14 per employee per month.

Benefit Design

The benefit is written in such a way as to discourage the use of inappropriate higher cost services and to encourage early intervention. For example, acute care hospitalization is authorized only for short-term crisis stabilization purposes, and structured outpatient (as opposed to inpatient or residential) rehabilitation programs are the rule for most patients who have not received previous treatment for drug or alcohol dependency. Outpatients seeing network providers are not asked to share any cost (co-payment) for the first five sessions.

The benefit also includes financial incentives and penalties aimed at both patients and providers to shape utilization in the direction of cost-effectiveness. Though they pay no co-payment for the first five sessions, outpatients pay an increasing amount as the number of sessions increase. They pay $5 per session for sessions 6–10, $10 per session for sessions 11–15, and $15 per session thereafter. If the patient chooses to receive outpatient services from a non-network provider, and if that provider is willing to cooperate with the case management system, the plan pays 50% of the negotiated fee for that service. The patient must pay the difference between that amount and the charged amount.

Patients receiving inpatient, residential, or a structured program of services (e.g., outpatient chemical dependency program; day treatment) in an organized care setting pay a 10% co-payment if the services are preauthorized and received from a network provider. If the services are for chemical dependency, however, and the patient does not complete the formal rehabilitative treatment program, the reimbursement is reduced by 50%. If the services are received in a non-network institution or program which participates in the case management activity, reimbursement is limited to 50% of the negotiated network rate for that type of program. The patient must pay the balance of the charged fee. In the case of either inpatient or outpatient services received from a non-network provider who refuses to participate with case management, the patient receives no reimbursement for services.

Other Conditions of the Agreement

The XYZ Corporation is concerned not only with the costs of the services they purchase for their employees and families, but also with the quality and outcome of these services. Hence, XYZ has negotiated with ABC for quarterly reports which provide empirical data concerning those aspects of the service which the XYZ managers believe are indicators of quality. These reports include data such as:

- Percent of patients entering alcohol and drug rehabilitation programs who complete them.
- Percent of patients unexpectedly readmitted to any structured program, residential, or inpatient facility.

- Mean patient satisfaction ratings for various types of care, problem types, and providers.
- Mean level of functioning at follow-up.
- Patient satisfaction with ABCs administrative services.

ABC and XYZ have agreed that as the managed care company increases the scope and sophistication of its information management system, the reports to XYZ also will expand to include a greater range of data. For example, ABC will add a standardized level of functioning scale for selected patients to be administered at the beginning and at termination of treatment.

PROVIDER PROFILING. ABC maintains a computer-based data system which is used to monitor utilization and other characteristics of service. This is the source, for example, of the quality reports provided to XYZ as part of their service contract. A primary objective of the data system is to allow ABC to develop "profiles" of individual and institutional providers so that ABC can make decisions about who should be removed from the network, who should be retained (and perhaps given additional responsibilities), and who needs additional professional development and other support in order to assure the quality of services desired by ABC. Data incorporated into the profiles include, but are not limited to:

- Average outpatient number of sessions.
- Average inpatient length of stay.
- Unplanned readmissions.
- Percent of patients completing treatment.
- Utilization of second opinions.
- Change score on appropriate scales from admission to discharge.
- Measure of patient satisfaction.
- Case manager ratings of provider clinical skill.

With respect to the quality of ABC's case management process, regular staff conferences target system inadequacies and identify needed improvements in utilization review and provider support. A formal system also monitors the clinical and service performance of case managers.

A Closer Look at Financing Structures

Under a health benefit plan, whether a traditional indemnity model or some form of managed care, two critical functions must be carried out: *administration of the plan* and *assumption of financial risk.* In addition, if the system is managed, some entity must *perform the case management function.*

Under traditional, non-managed, indemnity insurance plans, the insurance company was the entity to both bear the risk and administer the plan. In the 1980s, when a number of very large employers undertook to self-insure for their employees' health care, the risk shifted to them from the insurance company. Employers still had to contract with insurance companies (or independent third party administrators) to administer the benefit plan, however, since they had no expertise in this area. Such arrangements were called "administrative services only" (ASO) contracts. Most of these plans were not managed, and any case review by the insurance companies was generally retrospective, conducted on an *ad hoc* basis, and largely uninformed by expertise in mental health treatment.

When managed care companies entered the market, employers contracted with these companies to oversee their employees' utilization of services and used third-party administrators on an ASO basis. Under this type of arrangement, the financial risk remained with the employer. As the managed care companies became more experienced, however, they became eager to assume the risk themselves. Arrangements such as this were potentially more profitable for the managed care companies and also gave them better control of the provider system, since they were the purchasers. It is now common for managed care companies to bear the risk for contracts which they undertake.

Figure 1 provides a schematic representation of three typical models of financing, administration, and management, showing the locus of each function within each model. The top table in this figure represents the traditional non-managed indemnity plan. The middle table represents a managed self-insured plan which uses an insurance company to pay claims. The table at the bottom of the page represents a model in which a managed care company provides all three functions for a capitated fee per employee per month. This model is similar to that discussed in the ABC/XYZ example. Under this arrangement the cost for behavioral health services to the employer is a fixed amount per employee per month. If it costs ABC more than this amount to provide the services, the company must absorb the loss; if it costs less, ABC may keep the excess. ABC bears the financial risk through some risk vehicle. ABC also conducts the management of the cases.

It is important to note that Figure 1 is not exhaustive. There are many more variations of the administration-financing-management model. For example, many insurance companies now directly manage services.

Figure 1

Locus of Claims Administration, Case Management, and Risk Bearing in Three Common Types of Financing Arrangements

Traditional Purchased Indemnity Plan

	Claims Administration	Service Management	Risk Bearing
Insurance Company	X		X
Employer			
Case Management Organization			

Self-Insured Managed Program

	Claims Administration	Service Management	Risk Bearing
Insurance Company	X		
Employer			X
Case Management Organization		X	

Capitated Case Managed Program
(See Text)

	Claims Administration	Service Management	Risk Bearing
Insurance Company			
Employer			
Case Management Organization	X	X	X

SYSTEM LIMITATIONS, CONTROVERSIES, AND CHALLENGES

Managed care has been subject to some telling criticism, primarily by the provider community but also by consumers and consumer groups, many of whom consider it an inappropriate intrusion into practice and little more than an access-denying and cost-saving mechanism (DeLeon, Uyeda, & Welch, 1985). The following section highlights issues which tend to generate the most controversy and those which present the biggest challenges to the continued development of managed care in behavioral health services.

Confidentiality

Accountability requirements of third parties payers always bring with them requests for clinical information. As a consequence, it is generally accepted that a consumer who accepts third party coverage for health services has, de facto, sacrificed absolute confidentiality in the patient-provider relationship.

The information required of managed systems greatly exceeds what was generally requested for the adjudication of claims in traditional third-party insurance programs. It is no surprise, then, that consumers and providers express fears about managed care companies having access to such large amounts of information of such a sensitive nature. While the abuses of information predicted in the past have not materialized (e.g., see Shueman & Penner, 1988), many people still believe that managed care companies are incapable of guaranteeing the appropriate use of information, particularly if it is entered into a computerized data base which may be accessed by large numbers of people. Managed care organizations, for their part, have developed strict protocols for handling "hard copy" data and sophisticated data systems employing passwords, coding systems, special telephone lines, etc. to help ensure the security of computerized data.

Impact on the Therapeutic Relationship

The therapeutic relationship traditionally has been the most sacrosanct aspect of mental health services. According to theorists, the "bonding" (Sharfstein, 1991) between the patient and the therapist is the critical variable in the therapeutic process. Critics of managed care claim that the intrusion of the managed care representative, by threatening the essential confidentiality of the relationship and by bringing into question the professional autonomy and judgment of the provider, jeopardizes the bonding process and diminishes therapeutic effect.

There is no doubt that the case management process has some effect on the clinical relationship. Anecdotal reports from both patients and providers indicate that the introduction of case management, in at least some cases, is perceived as negative and as having a negative effect on the therapeutic process. The argument made by case management firms is that the positive contributions of the management process far outweigh any potential negative effects, and the net effect on treatment outcome is positive. Whether and how much the management process affects the relationship, and how any effects become manifest in treatment outcome, are a few of the many questions about managed care which must be addressed by programs of research and evaluation.

Impact on the Cost and Quality of Care

When case management programs were relatively new, the focus of service contracts was generally on cost. This limited focus was rightly criticized by providers, consumers, and employers. More recently, managed care companies have aspired to a more balanced approach in which quality is granted an enhanced status in the contracts.

While there is some evidence that managed care can result in reduced cost of particular types of behavioral health care, such as high cost inpatient cases, there is little evidence as to its longer term effect on cost in a service system (Darling, 1991). There is even less empirical evidence about the effect of case management on the quality of care, other than "raising the quality floor," by eliminating a proportion of the more egregious examples of poor quality service.

A significant challenge facing the managed care industry is to implement research and evaluation efforts to answer these cost and quality questions (VandenBos, 1993). Appropriate research and evaluation techniques have generally not been applied to managed care, but attempts to address these questions must be given the highest priority in all managed care companies. Research must address the questions in a comprehensive manner, including attention to factors as diverse as the financial cost to providers of complying with the management process and the less well-defined cost to employers if employees perceive case management as something which interferes with their access to preferred services.

Questions of Bias

Many members of the provider community have claimed that the bias within managed care programs against high intensity, longer term treatment sometimes contributes to inappropriate care being provided to a patient. Commentaries on managed care often contain examples of patients who were poorly served by these programs. The most typical example is that of the severely disabled patient, usually referred to as "treatment resistant," for whom long periods of hospitalization may yield very little apparent change. Such patients may be able to function outside of a 24-hour inpatient setting with the support of appropriate and effective community-based treatment programs, but these programs are often not available. In a typical scenario with a patient such as this, the managed care representative suggests discharge from inpatient care because of lack of progress. The provider argues that a few more months in the hospital will allow the patient to develop the skills necessary to be maintained in the community with the supports available there.

Another type of "poorly served" patient is the one who is seriously deficient in the basic skills required to cope with the normal stresses of daily living. In clinical parlance, this type of patient has a poorly differentiated ego. He or she is vulnerable to the ordinary events of life and typically ends up in a long term (over many years) treatment relationship which may take on a supportive or "maintenance" aspect. In a typical scenario for this type of case, the provider suggests that a very long term weekly, or more frequent, supportive outpatient relationship should be maintained. The managed care company suggests that the treatment regime become periodic with sessions scheduled during times of increased stress.

Careful analysis of such cases, however, indicate that the problems may be associated with one or more of the following: poor performance by the managed care organization; unreasonable expectations or ignorance on the part of the provider; and a lack of appropriate, high quality service alternatives in the community. A prime challenge to managed care companies is the development of protocols and procedures needed **routinely** to deal with these complex cases. A second is for such companies to use their influence to facilitate the development of appropriate community-based alternatives to serve the needs of the more severely disabled patients. Purchasers, providers, and managed care companies must, in concert, clarify the purposes of private benefit programs and determine appropriate strategies for providing for those patients whose needs can not appropriately be covered by the necessarily limited benefit. Such a debate would need to include consideration of how benefit programs can be complemented by the community mental health system. A concerted advocacy effort would seem to be critical in this regard.

Absence of Standards for Managed Care Companies

Providers, particularly those in inpatient settings, point to the practical problems involved in communicating with managed care organizations and satisfying their requests for information. Providers frequently claim that managed care personnel are often difficult to reach by phone and that their requests for information and the time line imperatives invoked are often unreasonable. It is also claimed that review and case management personnel perform their jobs poorly due to inadequate training, lack of clinical competence and sensitivity, or minimal experience with the types of care they are reviewing.

With so many managed care companies either new or rapidly expanding, it is to be expected that the quality of their policies and the performance of their staff would vary greatly. It is also to be expected that, in a marketplace where competition is not exclusively based on price, the quality will improve gradually as a result of feedback from patients, providers, and purchasers. Nonetheless, many informed observers believe that adequate solutions to the "quality of case management" problems will not be forthcoming without some kind of national initiatives to regulate these companies. While some states have undertaken to develop such regulations, most of the major companies conduct business across many states. Hence, a national strategy would seem to be necessary.

Financial Incentive to Deny Care

A major concern is that if a managed care company is allowed to assume the financial risk for a benefit plan, the company will have an incentive to deny care inappropriately to realize a larger profit. To deal with this potential problem, increasingly sophisticated purchasers are demanding comprehensive data describing services utilized by their employees so that quality may be monitored. It is argued, however, that such scrutiny is inadequate, since purchasers often do not have the experience or knowledge base to ask the correct questions, judge the adequacy of the data provided, or reasonably interpret the data. Clearly, however, an employer concerned about these issues can avail itself of the expertise required to make reasonable judgments. This may be in the form of in-house staff—for example, many employers have in-house employee assistance programs—or external consultants.

Legal Liability

It has been traditionally held that, since the decisions of third party payers affect payment rather than services, payers could not be held legally liable for an adverse outcome to a patient whose care they refused to reimburse (for example, a patient discharged from a hospital who subsequently committed suicide because a third party payer refused continued funding). The justification for this position was that it is the provider who has the "duty of care"—the responsibility to do what is necessary to ensure the welfare of a patient, regardless of the payment situation. A recent court decision in California (Carveth, 1990) suggests that this position may no longer be tenable. In the case in question, the judge's opinion was that, because of financial realities, denying payment was the equivalent of denying treatment. On that basis, the judge ordered a trial to proceed and focus on the issue of the clinical appropriateness of the third-party payer's decision that continued inpatient care was not necessary. This decision suggests that increasing control of the services sought by managed care companies brings with it a concomitant responsibility for the welfare of the beneficiary population.

Theoretical Basis of Care Management

Virtually all managed care organizations have proprietary sets of practice guidelines or criteria which describe appropriate use of particular types of services and empirically supported treatment of specified disorders. Until recently the contents of these criteria sets were known only to case management personnel. Accordingly, providers were being judged by criteria of which they had no knowledge. As a result of criticisms from providers and a change in attitude on the part of managed care firms, most of these companies have now published their criteria. What is necessary now is for the managed care industry to reach a consensus on a standard set of criteria which reflect the "best current practice," that is, empirically derived knowledge about treatment efficacy, and which can be used throughout the country. This national criteria set should be subject to continual review and revision based on both experience with application of the criteria in managed care programs and improvements in the knowledge base.

CONCLUSION

Sharfstein (1992) argues that the development of managed care is a direct result of the failure of the traditional health care financing system. Yet, clearly, it is also a consequence of the failure of professional mental health training programs to engender attitudes of accountability, of the professions themselves to adopt an appropriate accountability stance, and of the publicly funded research community systematically to forge process-outcome linkages.

It is generally easier to identify problems than to find effective solutions. In the case of behavioral health services, the solutions must address the complexity of causes both within and external to the service system. Two things appear to be true about the managed care models developed to date. The first is that they solve some of the more obvious problems while, as is clear from the previous discussion, creating new ones which themselves require solutions. The second is that they have, to date, fallen far short of providing the means for dealing with the fundamental failings in professional training, professional accountability, and mental health services research which manifestly contribute to the problems in the service system.

Certainly, one of the biggest challenges to managed care companies is to diminish the adversarial nature of the relationships which they have developed with service providers. Effective solutions to cost and quality problems will require open and sustained collaboration and cooperation between payers and providers. An indicator of the maturity of the industry would surely be an industry initiative proposing a series of national conferences focused on the types of the issues discussed in this chapter. The reward for such an initiative would be a partnership which would benefit the industry and provider communities as well as other stakeholders, including consumers, their families, and carers.

REFERENCES

Asher, J. (1981). *Assuring Quality Mental Health Services: The CHAMPUS Experience.* (ADM81-1099). Washington, DC: U.S. Government Printing Office.

Bent, R.J. (1988). Education for quality assurance. In G. Stricker and A.R. Rodriguez (Eds.), *Handbook of Quality Assurance in Mental Health.* New York: Plenum, 103–136.

Carveth, B.W. (1990, August 30). Wilson v. Blue Cross of Southern California et al. *Medical Benefits.*

Darling, H. (1991). Employers and managed care: What are the early returns? *Health Affairs, 10*(4), 147–160.

DeLeon, P.H., Uyeda, M.K., & Welch, B.L. (1985). Psychotherapy and HMOs: New partnership or new adversary? *American Psychologist, 40,* 1122–1124.

Englund, M.J. & Vaccaro, V.A. (1991). New systems to manage mental health care. *Health Affairs, 10,* 129–137.

Goldman, H.H., Adler, D.A., Berlant, J., et al (1993). The case for a services-based approach to payment for mental illness under National Health Care Reform. *Hospital and Community Psychiatry, 6,* 542–544.

Koch, A.L. (1988). Financing health services. In S.J. Williams & P.R. Torrens (Eds.), *Introduction to Health Services* (3rd Edition). New York: John Wiley & Sons.

Sharfstein, S.S. (1992). Managed mental health care. In A. Tasman & A.B. Riba (Eds.), *Review of Psychiatry,* Volume 11. Washington, DC: American Psychiatric Press, Inc., 570–584.

Shueman, S.A., & Penner, N.R. (1988). Administering a national program of mental health peer review. In G. Stricker and A.R. Rodriguez (Eds.), *Handbook of Quality Assurance in Mental Health.* New York: Plenum, 441–454.

VandenBos, G.R. (1993). U.S. mental health policy: Proactive evolution in the midst of health care reform. *American Psychologist, 48,* 283–290.

Vaughan, E.J. (1986). *Fundamentals of Risk and Insurance* (4th Edition). New York: John Wiley & Sons.

Chapter 2

THE ROAD FROM PEER REVIEW TO
MANAGED CARE: HISTORICAL PERSPECTIVE

NORMAN R. PENNER

W hile organized medicine as a whole has been resistant to managed
health care with its perceived emphasis on utilization review (UR)
and cost containment, those in the psychiatric community appear to
have been especially resistant and mistrustful. At the same time, providers in the allied mental health professions, including psychology and
social work, have displayed a consistent, reactive negativism to calls for
accountability, both within and external to the profession.

Such an attitude is somewhat ironic in view of the fundamental role of
the two major mental health professions in the development of a national
program which was the earliest predecessor of current managed behavioral
health systems. This chapter describes that program and highlights its
general promise in providing the professions with a meaningful opportunity to shape the development of both public and private behavioral
health service delivery systems while satisfying their responsibility for
public accountability. The chapter further describes the associations'
failure in their stewardship of this program, and their resultant loss of
influence in shaping current managed care systems.

THE PIONEERING ROLE OF THE CHAMPUS PROGRAM

In the U.S. the role of the federal and state governments in the
provision or financing of health care has generally been limited to the
poor and the physically or mentally handicapped. State governments
have typically had the greater responsibility, in keeping with the interpretation of the U.S. Constitution that activities and powers not specifically delegated to the Federal Government are retained by the states.

The allocation of responsibility for health care to the states minimized
the involvement of the federal government in this arena until the

mid-1950s. At that time the federal government promulgated a major health benefit program which was ultimately to have a significant influence on the way the insurance industry regarded coverage for mental and emotional conditions.

On June 7, 1956, President Eisenhower signed into law a program originally called the Military Medicare Program, but now known as the Civilian Health and Medical Program of the Uniformed Services, or CHAMPUS (van Dyke & Elliott, 1969). This program provided financing for medical care of dependents of active duty military personnel. It was, however, restricted to hospital care and excluded coverage for chronic or mental conditions. Given the nature of the beneficiary population and their political importance during the period of the Korean police action, however, the CHAMPUS law was liberalized (PL 89-614) ten years after it was promulgated.

The amendments expanded CHAMPUS coverage to include "nervous and mental" disorders and allowed coverage of unrestricted inpatient and outpatient psychiatric care. They also broadened the entitlement provisions of the program by including certain retirees and their dependents, and all dependents of deceased military personnel.

The impact of these changes was to significantly enlarge the pool of CHAMPUS beneficiaries as well as to expand the types of services the program covered. The combined result was an increase in the volume of business under the program from 650,000 claims and $70 million in fiscal year 1966 to more than 1.5 million claims and $160 million two years later (van Dyke & Elliott, 1969). The cost of the program continued to rise exponentially for the next three years.

The 1966 amendments became a significant factor in the expansion of third party coverage for mental illness and, ultimately, the development of UR and quality assurance programs in mental health care. At the time of their implementation they set CHAMPUS distinctly apart from other federal, and many private, benefit programs.

In the mid-1960s, the United States was the only western industrialized nation which did not have a national health program. Continued Congressional interest in national health insurance legislation in the following decade resulted in the introduction of a number of bills, but most of them provided very little in the way of coverage for mental illness. This was true also of the Medicare program, which had been authorized by the Social Security Amendments of 1965.

The reluctance on the part of Congress to include such coverage under

Medicare or any of the proposed national health insurance schemes was due primarily to two factors. First, they ascribed to the principle that the federal government would not provide benefits for a service which was covered by another entity. In the case of services for mental illness, they had traditionally been provided by states, in state institutions. A more critical factor was the fear among members of Congress about the potential cost of coverage for mental illness. Its various definitions were so broad that, by some estimates, 35%–40% of the population could fall into the mentally ill category (Srole, et al, 1962). Furthermore, experience had shown that as the number of providers grew, so did the population defined as mentally ill.

Private Sector Experience Providing Mental Health Coverage

In general, the early private health insurance programs offered little if anything in the way of coverage for mental health services. In the early to mid-1950s, however, several of the largest insurance companies began to offer "major medical" coverage which included outpatient care for mental disorders covered on the same basis as all other conditions—that is, reimbursing 75% or 80% of the charge and with no special limitations on fees, number of visits, or maximum dollar expenditures. The experience under these policies, however, was that total charges for outpatient psychiatric care constituted an unacceptably high proportion of physicians' charges for all conditions. Moreover, some large claims for outpatient psychoanalysis and other long-term psychotherapies were submitted by beneficiaries who were not disabled or hospitalized, and who were holding down responsible jobs and earning sizeable incomes. These charges for services were submitted under benefit programs which were intended to restore disabled persons to an adequate level of functioning. The realization that they were paying significant amounts of benefit dollars, not for restoration, but for "self-improvement" and "self-knowledge" among a relatively small number of non-disabled persons who seemed to be functioning very effectively while undergoing treatment, prompted the companies to search for mechanisms to ensure that benefits for mental health treatment would be equitably consumed.

An example of the efforts to gain some control occurred in the late 1950s in context of the health insurance program covering New York State employees. Coverage under the state plan included a major medical supplement which provided for payment of 75% of covered charges after a deductible; the same condition held for both mental and other conditions. Major medical claims for outpatient psychiatric care for the state employees were much greater than anticipated, and the insurance company asked a committee of psychiatrists to review the claims experience. The review revealed that the greater portion of the outpatient psychiatric claims expense was for psychoanalysis, much of it for training analysis for psychiatrists working at the state mental hospitals. A significant number of claims also came from social workers at the state hospitals and in the State Department of Social Welfare who undertook psychoanalysis as a means of enhancing their prospects for job advancement. Based on these findings, the insurance companies drastically reduced benefits for outpatient psychiatric care (Reed, Myers, & Scheidemandel, 1972) and, as word of their experience spread throughout the insurance industry, the practice of setting specific limits on psychiatric benefits was adopted by other companies. By the mid-1960s, the practice had become an industry standard.

There were two rather significant exceptions to the practice of setting arbitrary limits. The first was in the CHAMPUS program described above. The second was in the Government-Wide Indemnity Benefit Plan, offered by a consortium of insurance companies under the direction of AEtna Life & Casualty Company to federal employees under the Federal Employees Health Benefits Program. While CHAMPUS provided unlimited coverage for both inpatient and outpatient psychiatric care, AEtna (in 1971) covered mental and nervous disorders, in or out of hospital, on the same basis as all other illnesses. However, both of these programs began to experience significant adverse utilization in their coverage of mental conditions.

Federal Initiatives to Control Cost and Quality

Following the amendments of 1966, not only did the total cost of CHAMPUS continue to grow, but the percent of total CHAMPUS disbursements covering mental health also grew disproportionately. To add to the program's problems, it was rocked by a scandal in 1974 involving residential treatment of emotionally disturbed children.

The extraordinary cost overruns of the program attracted the attention of the House Armed Services Committee during the budget preparation cycle of 1968–69, and the Committee directed the General Accounting Office (GAO) to conduct a series of audits of CHAMPUS. The residential treatment scandal drew the attention of the Senate Government Operations Committee's Permanent Subcommittee on Investigations which held a series of public hearings (Asher, 1981).

The early 1970s were difficult ones for CHAMPUS. Government scrutiny revealed that the program had significant deficiencies in both cost and quality. Testimony before the Senate Committee revealed shocking abuses of adolescent CHAMPUS beneficiaries. The GAO audits found that the CHAMPUS program was being poorly administered generally and, more specifically, that the mental health benefits had come to include a far wider scope than Congress had intended. The GAO's fourth and final report of its audits of CHAMPUS was devoted entirely to the subject of mental health coverage under the program. This report was issued in 1972 and was followed by a reorganization of CHAMPUS management within the Department of Defense (DoD). The most significant step was to take responsibility for the management of the program away from the Surgeon General of the Army and set up a special office within the Office of the Assistant Secretary of Defense for Health Affairs at the Pentagon. This office was established in late 1972 and its staff immediately began working on resolutions to the problems cited in the GAO reports.

Government Overtures to the Professions

The cost and coverage issues relative to the mental health benefits were addressed initially by establishing a dialogue with the American Psychiatric Association and the American Psychological Association, the two major mental health professional organisations in the U.S. These overtures were welcomed by both associations, as CHAMPUS was recognized to be a model benefits program (i.e., was generous with regard to payment for mental health treatment) and was often cited as such by the associations when they "lobbied" other third-party payers.

The American Psychiatric Association was receptive to an opportunity to work with the DoD/CHAMPUS officials because its membership had become very concerned about the growing restrictions the major insurance carriers were placing on mental health coverage. The association had just put significant, unsuccessful, effort into attempts to open up the Medicare program to broader psychiatric benefits, and they saw the CHAMPUS relationship as an important one to ensure that the program's excellent benefits were maintained. The Psychological Association shared the enthusiasm of the psychiatrists, but they had an additional reason for welcoming the overture: it was seen as an all-too-rare example of being accorded "parity" with psychiatry.

The Psychiatric Association had previously demonstrated its commitment to public accountability in context of the Federal Medicare Program. In that case the Association's efforts had been precipitated by the newly mandated Professional Services Review Organizations (PSROs) which were organized to monitor hospital care for Medicare and Medicaid. The federal law mandating these organizations also contained authorization for monitoring ambulatory care. The American Medical Association (AMA), attempting to take some initiative in the way the PSROs would operate, requested that all professional medical organizations develop model review criteria and then submit them to the AMA which would, in turn, make the criteria available to the government for use by the PSROs. Organized psychiatry saw the request for development of criteria as providing an opportunity for the APA to represent itself as a responsible and accountable professional organization. This association was the first and only professional medical organization to commit itself to the development of and actually deliver the requested model criteria.

The residential treatment crisis in CHAMPUS also provided the mental health community an opportunity to publicly demonstrate a commitment to accountability as they participated with the DoD in efforts to improve quality. In response to the Senate hearings, the Deputy Assistant Secretary of Defense for Health Resources and Programs wrote Senator Jackson, majority chairman of the Senate Subcommittee, that coverage of psychiatric treatment had been a relatively uncontrolled element of the CHAMPUS program. He cited lack of standards and monitoring as major failures which were rooted, in part, in the prevailing philosophy that any care legitimized by a physician's signature should be reimbursed. He pointed out also that the quality assurance plan then being conceptualized to correct the residential treatment situation would provide an appropriate model for dealing with problems in other CHAMPUS-covered psychiatric program areas.

The quality assurance plan referred to in the letter to Senator Jackson was the product of discussions between DoD staff and staff of the National Institute of Mental Health (NIMH). The two organizations had reached an agreement that NIMH would establish, and DoD would fund, a panel of nationally recognized mental health professionals to investigate the problems in residential treatment. This panel, called the Select Committee on Psychiatric Care and Evaluation (SCOPCE), was established in

October of 1974. It consisted of teams of independent consultants (psychiatrists, psychologists, social workers, and psychiatric nurses) whose responsibilities were to review records of treatment of the 500 child and adolescent CHAMPUS beneficiaries then in residential treatment centers, and to make judgments about the appropriateness of the placements, the quality of care, and the appropriateness of length of stay and costs (Asher, 1981).

By the summer of 1977 when it concluded its work, SCOPCE had reviewed some 1,500 cases at a cost of about $250,000. An actuarial study based on 800 cases reviewed during the first phase of the project estimated the savings at more than $5 million. SCOPCE nearly halved the cost of the residential treatment benefit during its first year of operation, cutting it from $13.2 million in 1974 to $7.8 million in 1975.

Benefits to the Profession from the SCOPCE Effort

Since the American Psychiatric Association was given a significant leadership role in the SCOPCE project, that association garnered a significant amount of good will and positive publicity for its efforts. As a result, the concept of professional (peer) review as an alternative to the more draconian absolute limits became favored by the Psychiatric Association leadership, and it strongly encouraged its state organizations (district branches) to appoint Peer Review Committees. These committees were to establish contact with local representatives of insurance companies and offer their services to review troublesome cases. Organized psychology had similar committees, called Professional Services Review Committees, organized through the state psychological associations.

While insurance companies saw the value of local review in accommodating the generally accepted "local standards" of practice, the national carriers preferred to deal with one entity rather than with 70 district branches and 50 state associations. Despite this fact, several of the major carriers did attempt to utilize the local organizations. Of particular importance were the attempts by AEtna Life & Casualty.

AEtna's effort, under the direction of William Guillette, Medical Director for Group Health Plans, had been relatively unsuccessful due primarily to two factors. First, not all district branches nor state psychological associations had appointed committees, and, second, among those that did, the groups were often non-responsive and sometimes even hostile. For example, in Washington, D.C., an area particularly problematic for AEtna's Federal Employee Health Benefits Program, the chairman of the district branch committee accused AEtna of being "on a fishing expedition," looking for reasons to deny psychiatric claims. Guillette informed the associations that, as a result of their apparent inability to be responsive to AEtna, company officials were planning to make significant reductions in coverage for mental and emotional conditions.

In the meantime, the discussions between the two national professional associations and CHAMPUS continued with no significant resolutions forthcoming. The associations' size, complexity, and need to acknowledge member interests precluded prompt ratification or approval of changes. Just as important, agreement between the two organizations was even more difficult than agreement within them. Given the lack of progress and the continued deterioration of CHAMPUS' fiscal situation, the Secretary of Defense decided, in the summer of 1974, to issue a public announcement of a number of significant changes to be implemented within the following six months. These plans included the institution of absolute limits on the mental health benefits similar to those being used by most commercial insurance carriers.

This announcement by the Secretary was a major shock to the mental health services provider community. They quickly found common ground and organized joint committees to lobby Congress and the Secretary of Defense. Patients were encouraged to write to their Congressional representatives and protest the proposed changes.

Since the U.S. was deeply involved in the Viet Nam conflict at the time, Congress faced a serious dilemma. On the one hand it had been pressuring CHAMPUS to reduce its costs, and the proposal to limit benefits was a response to the pressure. On the other hand, Congress did not want to be party to any activity that would be seen to reflect a lack of concern for the welfare of the members of the armed forces and their families.

At this point, all the participants were searching for a reasonable compromise. The representative of the Psychiatric Association suggested that CHAMPUS use peer review as an alternative to the proposed limits. He pointed out that the SCOPCE project was working very well and the mental health professionals participating in the project had clearly demonstrated a willingness to deal decisively with their professional colleagues when they discovered abuses. Furthermore, the use of professionals to police themselves would be far more palatable to providers and more equitable for patients than arbitrary limits, and it would be equally effective.

Seeing this as a reasonable compromise as well as a way out of their dilemma, DoD withdrew its plans to limit psychiatric benefits, with the understanding that the American Psychiatric Association would develop a "psychiatric peer review program" for CHAMPUS. As with the SCOPCE effort, DoD would underwrite the expense. Since CHAMPUS also paid for outpatient psychotherapy provided by psychologists, and because the two professions had a longstanding tacit agreement prohibiting members of one from reviewing work of members of the other, DoD was advised that it should offer the same opportunity to the American Psychological Association.

Thus, in 1977 the Department of Defense entered into agreements with both APAs. The contracts called for each association to develop a national peer review program for its constituency. Psychiatry had the task of developing a review program for all inpatient care and for outpatient psychiatric services. Psychology was to design a program for outpatient psychological services as well as psychological assessment. Both organizations appointed an oversight committee and proceeded to write criteria and protocols.

IMPLEMENTATION OF PEER REVIEW

Both professional associations began conducting reviews for CHAMPUS in early 1979. The initial contracts were for three years and, during the early years, many problems arose, some of which were never completely resolved. The projects gained significant public attention, however, and both associations gained favorable publicity from these activities.

The major insurance carriers increasingly consulted with the two associations' CHAMPUS advisory committees on policy issues and used the associations' reviewers to assist them in resolving difficult cases. In essence, these private companies were able to benefit from a "product"—a professional review service—the development of which was paid for by the federal government. The number of insurance companies using the services of the two organizations continued to increase. There was noticeable improvement in the attitudes of many of the major national carriers toward psychiatry and psychology as a result of the new responsiveness shown by the associations. Contact was established between the carriers and the professional associations' governance groups, and effective communication endured for several years.

Non-Mental Health Review Activity

In the late 1970s and early 1980s significant quality assurance and UR developments were also occurring in the non-psychiatric areas of medicine. The PSROs were in full operation by 1980, a time which also saw the advent of private review organizations in the medical-surgical arena. Second surgical opinions were a popular cost-containment innovation increasingly used by insurance companies. Case management also had its beginning in the disability insurance field during this period. Preadmission and concurrent review were beginning to replace the retrospective review of medical and surgical claims. None of the private review organizations, however, was conducting UR of mental health services. These services were considered by the companies to be too subjective and poorly defined. It was the system established by the two mental health professional associations for CHAMPUS that served as the vanguard for the development of a significant utilization review industry focused on behavioral health services.

Privatization of Care Management

In 1976 the American Psychiatric Association published a *Manual of Psychiatric Peer Review* (APA, 1976) which was initially intended to be used by its district branch peer review committees. The document remained unnoticed outside the profession until entrepreneurial psychiatrists and psychologists realized that there was a market for psychiatric UR and began setting up companies to provide these services. This manual became the foundation for in-house systems for some of these organizations, since it gave their efforts a creditable base. At the same time, the criteria themselves had little inherent value, based as they were on "usual and customary" practices (Shueman & Troy, 1994).

Prior to 1979, 17 utilization review vendors were operating in the U.S. Most of these companies reviewed disability cases or provided second surgical opinions, while a few had been performing some review of medical and surgical hospital admissions. The major growth in the number of UR vendors did not begin until 1982 when five new firms were founded. In 1985, 21 new UR vendors came into existence. By this time, most of the established UR vendors had added psychiatric and substance abuse review services to their standard products in response to clients' demands. They performed relatively simple modifications to

their medical and surgical review procedures and criteria to accommo-
date psychiatric admissions, and they usually used their existing in-house
staff to conduct the reviews.

One of the oldest UR vendors, Intracorp, realized that the review of
psychiatric and substance abuse admissions required specialized knowledge, and recognized that they did not have appropriate expertise in-house.
The strategy they adopted to deal with this problem was to enter into a
joint venture with the American Psychiatric Association. Under the
terms of this agreement, signed in 1983, the association's Office of Quality Assurance, which was responsible for the CHAMPUS contract, was to
conduct telephone-based preadmission and concurrent reviews of all
psychiatric admissions for Intracorp's clients. Through this arrangement,
Intracorp gained the expertise of an experienced psychiatric UR vendor
and, at the same time, capitalized on their formal affiliation with the
major mental health professional association.

The Professions Lose Influence

Although the American Psychiatric Association and the American
Psychological Association had been the pioneers in the managed mental
health field through their CHAMPUS and related review activities,
their efforts began to falter in the mid-1980s. From the outset, both
associations had significant membership opposition to the basic concept
of review, but the general level of acceptance was sufficient for the
programs to proceed. The acceptance was based on two factors. The first
was that the review program was presented as the only viable way of
retaining the very beneficial CHAMPUS program and overcoming some
of the negative perceptions of the mental health professions held by the
insurance industry and federal health policy makers. While there was a
good deal of rhetoric about assuring the quality of care delivered to
patients and concern over patient welfare, it is likely that large numbers
of members of both associations saw the review efforts primarily as a
means to protect their economic interests. The second factor affecting
acceptance was that, for a significant period of time after the associations
signed the agreements with CHAMPUS, clinicians were not actually
affected by the review program. Implementation did not begin for over
two years, and, when it finally did, it was phased in relatively slowly in
different parts of the country.

Significant exceptions to this cynicism about the review efforts existed within both associations among the general membership and, even more so, among those professionals who were involved in the development of the review systems and the hundreds of psychologists and psychiatrists who conducted the reviews. These persons saw the efforts as contributing to the betterment of the quality of patient care and, because of their efforts, both review programs flourished for five years.

The turning point for the two professions' review activities occurred in 1985 when DoD decided that it could no longer continue to contract with the two APAs under non-competitive terms, as it had been doing for almost nearly a decade. By this time, there were other well established UR vendors who also sought the opportunity to bid on the CHAMPUS business. The government suggested, however, that if the two associations were to enter into a joint venture, it might be able to justify continuing to use them on a non-competitive basis. This suggestion resulted in an unsuccessful attempt by the two associations to negotiate a joint venture. Their inability to agree on terms resulted in the government soliciting competitive bids for the peer review activity. The two associations were among the bidders, and the Psychiatric Association was the victor.

Psychology's Withdrawal from Review

The Psychological Association's failure to win the contract was no doubt related to the Psychiatric Association's traditional dominance in the behavioral health services field. A contributing factor, however, was probably the organization's insistence on viewing the review program as a vehicle for advocacy. The association's submission to CHAMPUS integrated proposals for restructuring certain aspects of the CHAMPUS benefit to eliminate those conditions which psychologists found most abhorrent. For example, the CHAMPUS regulation gave ultimate authority for treatment, and therefore review, in inpatient settings to physicians, even if that treatment was provided by a psychologist in a state where psychologists had "admitting privileges", or were given legal responsibility, in inpatient facilities. The Psychological Association proposed that CHAMPUS-funded services provided by a psychologist in a hospital be reviewed by psychologists. As a result of such provisions the association's proposal was regarded as partially non-responsive to CHAMPUS's request for proposal.

This advocacy position was partly to mollify the growing number of psychologists who had developed negative attitudes about third party review. Review activities by this time had been adopted by almost all major insurers, and mental health providers were feeling increasingly burdened by the process. A former director of the psychological CHAMPUS project provided one perspective on the attitude of the association at that time:

> Unfortunately, many psychologists practicing in the field and not aware of the political implications (or more concerned with their own immediate welfare) saw little if any advocacy function in the peer review program. It was seen only as taking things away from the independent practitioner. And, clearly [in their view], the association could not simultaneously advocate for psychologists and participate in a system which intruded on their therapeutic relationship and took money out of the pockets of practitioners (Shueman, 1987).

This assessment of the psychologists would prove to be equally applicable to psychiatrists three years later.

Psychiatry's Withdrawal from Review

During the three year period following the successful bid to conduct review of all mental health services, the psychiatric UR program prospered, generating over $18.5 million in revenues and adding some $2.2 million to the APA's assets. These economic facts contributed to the support for the program within the association's governance.

The demise of the psychiatric program began in 1988 when Intracorp terminated its agreement with the APA. This came about for several reasons. First, there was a slight downturn in Intracorp's financial growth and, in the view of many, the company became conservative in its outlook. The APA leadership, on the other hand, was convinced of the APA's unique value to Intracorp's continued success in the UR industry. Believing that this gave them significant leverage with Intracorp, the association requested changes to the contract between the two organizations. Intracorp, for its part, believed it had learned enough about psychiatric UR to conduct independent psychiatric review, and terminated the relationship with the APA.

APA's loss of the Intracorp business was followed by their loss of the CHAMPUS contract. The contract had again been put out for competitive bidding, and, for this bid cycle, numerous private sector review organizations were both capable of conducting the program and eager for the business. At the same time, the government no longer believed they needed the imprimatur of the major mental health professional association for the UR program to have credibility and to be accepted by providers. The result of the bidding process was that the CHAMPUS contract was awarded to a private review company, Health Management Strategies.

After the dissolution of the joint venture with Intracorp, the APA organized its own company, Advanced PsychSystems (APS), through which it continued to market UR services. A marketing program was underway at the time the APA was competing for the CHAMPUS contract, and projections were for APS to be financially viable within 12–18 months. The loss of the CHAMPUS contract, however, combined with the phenomenal growth of the private psychiatric review industry combined to turn the tide of support within the association away from the review program and ensure the demise of APS.

Membership displeasure with the increasing demands of UR vendors was growing, and members were putting increasing pressures on their association to take concerted action against these companies. The association could not publicly oppose UR while operating its own UR company. At the same time, the review program no longer looked like the economic asset that it had been in the days of the CHAMPUS and Intracorp contracts. Thus, in late 1989, the American Psychiatric Association formally withdrew from the review business.

The Current Status

By the end of 1989, the two major professional associations had handed over entirely to the private, for-profit business community the cost and quality management of behavioral health services. Closing remarks at the 1987 meeting of the psychologists by that association's former CHAMPUS Project Director were now equally appropriate for the psychiatrists:

> The Association's disinclination to pursue review significantly reduced its potential role in structuring both publicly- and privately-funded "managed" mental health care systems. Such systems, which will inevitably dominate mental health delivery for the next decade, all have as critical elements some type of review program demanding of providers adherence to carefully conceived treatment plans. To a very great extent, these programs are currently being fashioned without the input of organized psychology. An open question for the profession is whether its withdrawal from the peer review arena was worth the cost it will bear in terms of loss of influence. More importantly, to the extent that the abandonment of the peer review program was an Association statement concerning the relative values of accountability versus guild

interests, a second important question for the profession is whether organized psychology needs to reconsider its apparent total commitment to guild-oriented advocacy (Shueman, 1987).

The two professional associations have seemingly come full circle in their involvement with professional services review. Having established for themselves a leadership role, they have withdrawn from the field. Where they were once active in setting criteria for determining medical and psychological necessity and judging quality, they have now chosen to resist further initiatives in managed care. Both associations have considered legal action to combat the activities of the managed care industry and have been engaged in lobbying for state legislation which would either regulate or prohibit managed care activities.

CONCLUSION

While the two professions seem to have abdicated what some would argue is their legitimate responsibility to participate in the shaping of behavioral health services review and delivery systems, many of the individual professionals involved in the development and implementation of these early review programs have continued their work, but in the private sector. In addition, many of these private organizations have used and built upon the protocols, procedures, and criteria developed by the associations during their decade of peer review activity.

Strong arguments have been made with regard to professional membership associations that there is an inherent conflict between guild interests and public interest. It is perhaps appropriate, then, not to lament the withdrawal of the mental health professions from the review arena, but rather to appreciate the fact that the two associations were involved in critical, formative stages when their influence over their members was of greatest importance.

REFERENCES

Asher, J. (1981). *Assuring quality mental health services: The CHAMPUS experience.* (ADM81-1099). Washington, D.C.: U.S. Government Printing Office.

Reed, L.S., Myers, E., & Scheidemandel, P.L. (1972). *Health Insurance and Psychiatric Care: Utilization and Cost.* Washington, DC: American Psychiatric Association.

Shueman, S. A. (1987). The professional association and peer review: Accountability versus advocacy. Paper presented at the annual meeting of the American Psychological Association, New York, August.

Shueman, S.A. & Penner, N.R. (1989). Administering a national program of mental health peer review. In G. Stricker & A. Rodriguez (Eds.), *Handbook of Quality Assurance in Mental Health.* New York: Plenum, 441–454.

Shueman, S.A. & Troy, W.G. (1994). Use of practice guidelines in managed behavioral health care programs. In S.A. Shueman, W.G. Troy, and S.L. Mayhugh (Eds.), *Managed Behavioral Health Care: An Industry Perspective.* Springfield, Illinois: Charles C Thomas, 149–163.

Srole, L., et al (1962). *Midtown Manhattan Study.* New York: McGraw-Hill.

van Dyke, F. & Elliott, R. (1969). Military Medicare. Report submitted to the Department of Defense by the School of Public Health, Columbia University, June.

PART II
MANAGED CARE IN PRACTICE:
NEW ROLES FOR CLINICIANS

PART II: INTRODUCTORY NOTE

Managed care requires professionals providing behavioral health services to adopt new roles and to modify significantly the way they work and the professional attitudes they embrace. In Chapter 3, Mayhugh and Shueman present a context for understanding these new roles by describing why and how managed care programs construct their networks, what kinds of professionals they look for and what kinds of behaviors they expect from them, their criteria for provider performance, and what network providers can expect in return from the managed care company.

As becomes clear in chapter 3, the significant challenge to providers relates to demands by managed care companies for changes in typical patterns of practice. While a majority of mental health professionals have been trained in non-directive, long-term or open-ended models of therapeutic intervention focused on change of personality structure, managed care programs require a structured, directive, time-limited approach focused on restoring patients to an adequate level of functioning.

Also difficult for professionals to accept is the managed care company's perspective on the therapeutic relationship, one in which the company is a significant participant. Under traditional reimbursement systems, payers requested little clinical information beyond a diagnosis. Even under these circumstances, however, providers submitted minimal information or expressed what they did submit in terms which were considered "non-stigmatizing". Managed programs require information which is sufficient to make decisions about necessity and appropriateness of services. That sharing of information of this scope and level of detail is demanded by managed care companies is perhaps, from the providers' perspective, the most objectionable aspect of managed care. Not only is it seen as a violation of the sanctity of the patient-provider relationship, it is also regarded as an inappropriate infringement on provider autonomy.

Not surprisingly, an often intense adversarial relationship exists between managed care programs and providers. As a consequence, many professionals focus their energies on defeating these systems and, thereby, increase the probability that the managed care process will have a detrimental effect on the clinical process. Such a stance also effectively eliminates any chance of providers playing a role in shaping managed systems.

In Chapter 4, Lane offers providers an alternative, more positive perspective, intended to empower and encourage them to take a more assertive stance with managed care companies. Based on the assumption that services management is here to stay for the foreseeable future, Lane suggests that professionals assume the role of a business person with a commodity to sell. This presupposes, of course, that providers know what they have to sell and want to sell it in the managed marketplace — two determinations which must be made through a process of honest and careful self-assessment. Lane also suggests that providers determine what they need from the managed care company and use this information to take a more active role in creating their own futures and in shaping the managed systems with which they work.

What is seldom acknowledged by providers dealing with managed care companies is that professionals responsible for implementing the case management process are mental health professionals just like themselves, often with very similar training and experiences, and with a similar commitment to service quality. Despite some claims to the contrary, case managers almost invariably report that their primary concerns are the necessity and appropriateness of services and that cost concerns are, while important, only secondary.

In Chapter 5, Reinhardt and Shepherd provide a personal perspective of mental health professionals who are the voices on the other end of the phone line in one very specialized case management organization. They attempt to give the reader some insight into the roles and responsibilities as they define them, as well as the frustration and gratification which they experience in their work. This presentation demonstrates clearly the potential for constructive collaboration which exists in a system characterized by a flexible benefit structure, staffed by competent case managers, and having network providers who view managed care personnel as resources rather than adversaries.

Chapter 3

THE DEVELOPMENT AND MAINTENANCE OF PROVIDER NETWORKS

BRIAN L. MAYHUGH AND SHARON A. SHUEMAN

An essential characteristic of a managed care program is a designated provider network, including both individual practitioners (usually psychiatrists, psychologists, clinical social workers, and marriage and family counselors) and organized care settings such as hospitals, residential treatment centers, and structured outpatient alcohol and drug rehabilitation programs. Network providers agree to offer treatment for a predetermined fee according to conditions established by the managed care company. They constitute a defined group of practitioners who, presumably, embrace the company's normative approach to service provision and ascribe to its accountability procedures.

This chapter deals with the substance and rationale of some of the major decisions involved in the development and maintenance of a provider network for a managed behavioral health care program. The primary emphasis is on individual providers. Consideration is given to recruitment and selection, as well as to network monitoring and improvement of provider performance.

The chapter describes what is, in some ways, a model network approach. For a variety of reasons, a number of managed care companies undertake the development and maintenance of networks in a much less systematic fashion than is depicted here. Such non-strategic approaches typically come from pressures to establish a network quickly, for example, in order to service a particular contract or to develop a sufficiently large network to satisfy a state regulatory requirement. Non-optimal development approaches may also occur with companies who claim little confidence in the utility of formal selection criteria for identifying the more desirable providers. Such companies initially select providers on an essentially random basis, subsequently retaining those whose practice patterns and outcomes conform to the companies' criteria for performance.

In this instance, the organization would use a minimal categorical set of qualifying criteria (such as possession of state license and evidence of liability insurance coverage) as the basis for initial selection, and then depend upon monitoring, feedback, and termination of unsatisfactory providers to achieve what is deemed to be an adequate level of service quality.

Non-systematic approaches too frequently characterize the maintenance of existing networks. Proper monitoring of provider practices and outcomes demands extra time on the part of case managers and other staff of the managed care company, and requires the use of a computer-based information system to develop and evaluate practice profiles. Monitoring is a resource-intensive activity which may be accorded low priority in the competition for financial and other resources within the managed care company. In the companies which accord network maintenance lower priority, corrective action is usually taken only in the case of obviously problematic providers.

Why a Network?

Managed care companies use designated networks to increase their control over the service system. The objective is to have access to a limited group of providers who are, in their collectivity, more competent than a randomly selected group would be, and who agree in advance to abide by requirements for accountability and ascribe to a particular service orientation. Careful selection and monitoring of provider performance are presumed to allow the company to achieve less variation in service quality than would occur in an uncontrolled fee-for-service system. The existence of a negotiated, generally discounted, fee structure also gives the company at least a modicum of control over service costs.

From a system perspective, identifiable networks have other advantages, primarily related to accessibility and continuity of care. For example, the existence of a network removes much of the uncertainty from the referral process conducted by case managers who know the pool of providers, where their offices are located, what services they provide, and what types of patients they typically serve. An identified network system also ensures availability of the necessary complement of appropriately credentialed service providers in any given geographic area. Finally, the use of a "gatekeeper" mechanism is designed to minimize patients' self-initiated and unconstrained use of multiple or potentially inappropriate service providers.

Opportunistic and non-strategic approaches to network development and maintenance will inevitably yield service systems whose quality can not be assured. Only through a careful process of selection, monitoring, feedback, professional development and retraining, and, ultimately, termination of those providers whose performance has failed to satisfy the designated criteria, can a company hope to achieve a network of high quality. An effective network is not, for example, what one large managed care company achieved by designating all licensed psychiatrists within a particular state as members. Nor is it what a second company secured by contracting almost exclusively with masters level providers because they would work for lower fees. Effective networks, once established, must constantly be re-fashioned. It is an exacting process and a costly one. No networks are ever "good enough."

Parameters of a Network

While a network consists of individual practitioners and programs, it is more usefully viewed as an entity or system. The adequacy of such a system is determined, in part, by the extent to which it satisfies criteria related to size, geographic coverage, and composition.

Network Size

The development of a provider network, if done well, involves a significant initial cost—direct and foregone. In addition, network maintenance involves appreciable recurrent costs. Lastly, the greater the number of providers, the more difficult it is for case managers to become familiar with them, their particular strengths, competencies, and needs. A prime objective of many managed care firms is, therefore, to optimize the size of the network so that it is no larger than necessary. It must be large enough to serve the needs of the enrolled populations and the benefit plans associated with beneficiaries. Once this size is assured, however, little purpose is served by an increase in the number of providers.

A secondary advantage in limiting the size of networks is that smaller networks result in a greater number of referrals and, hence, greater income for individual providers. Receiving a large number of referrals from a single managed care program is important if providers are expected to adhere to a strategic, time-limited service focus. If they can be assured

as to the continuity of a referral stream, network providers are likely to
have less motivation to extend the treatment of patients for whom they
are currently responsible. Having a large number of patients from a
particular company also acts to increase the provider's identification
with and commitment to that company—significant factors from a quality assurance perspective.

Geographic Coverage

Managed care companies are generally obligated to ensure that their
provider networks offer adequate geographic coverage. This is commonly interpreted to mean that an adequate number and mix of network
providers are located within a specified number of miles or driving time
of any given beneficiary. Requirements for coverage may be explicated
in state law or regulation applying to prepaid health plans or other
service delivery programs.

Companies also attempt to guarantee beneficiaries access to more than
a single network provider to enable them to exercise choice in the
selection of the person from whom they will receive services. It may not
be possible, however, to guarantee a meaningful choice for beneficiaries
who live in geographically isolated areas. In such situations, managed
care companies may induct providers into the network who do not satisfy
all of the company's own criteria for eligibility for network membership.
The company may even utilize non-network providers.

Provider Mix

There is significant overlap in the types of services which the different
mental health professions claim as part of their clinical repertoire and
which licensing authorities permit them to offer. Most significantly,
these provider groups all have the right to engage in and claim developed
expertise in individual psychotherapy. To some extent, then, representatives from different disciplines are treated by the managed care organization as interchangeable, given that the distribution of intervention skills
across the groups—rightly or wrongly—is not seen to be significantly
different. At the same time, there are obvious differences across providers and provider groups with regard to particular competencies which
are acquired either through training or experience, or are conferred
upon particular professions by virtue of the state licensing process. The
decision as to who should be selected for a network is commonly made

on the basis of need for particular competencies within the network, as well as on the basis of relative cost of providers.

THE COST OF PROVIDERS. Whether associated with managed systems or not, doctoral level practitioners command higher fees than those with lesser qualifications. It does not necessarily follow, however, that to rely primarily on providers with lesser qualifications is a cost-effective strategy. The relative cost of the various types of mental health professionals is a consideration in developing a network, but it is by no means the primary determiner of network composition. A lower-fee provider may have consistently poor outcomes, or may have cost-ineffective practice patterns, such as the tendency to prolong treatment or to utilize unnecessary clinical procedures. If two providers offering the same service are of equal competence with respect to that service, the less costly individual is, from the perspective of the service system, the better choice. In such a situation cost is a reasonable criterion for selection. If the more expensive provider is superior, however, then the question of preference from a system perspective has no easy answer and requires more careful analysis of cost-benefit issues.

SPECIALIST COMPETENCIES. Managed systems are primarily interested in generalist providers who can deal effectively with a majority of the problem and patient types typically seen in a comprehensive behavioral health service system. This aside, however, not all providers will be qualified or even willing to provide all services for all patient types. Consequently, the composition of the network is partially determined by a consideration of the range of specialist competencies needed within a geographic area by a particular beneficiary population.

There are several ways of conceptualizing competencies which are relevant to the process of selecting professionals for a network. The first relates to functions which are restricted to certain disciplines under *state licensing laws.* For example, psychiatrists may prescribe medication and may admit patients to hospitals. In certain jurisdictions, psychologists or even other professionals may have admitting privileges.

A second view of competencies focuses on those which belong to certain groups by virtue of their *discipline-specific professional training.* In theory, such services may be provided by any practitioner, but general expectations are that competence derives from discipline-specific professional training. An obvious example of such a specialty is psychological testing and assessment. All doctoral students in psychology learn these skills. Such skills are not generally a part of training in psychiatry or social work, even though some members of these disciplines do administer and interpret psychological tests. A second example of discipline-specific training is the treatment of psychological correlates of medical conditions (e.g., chronic pain, recovery from life-threatening illness), such as would be performed by psychologists trained in health psychology programs. By and large, managed care companies designate "appropriate" disciplines to be providers of these types of services.

A third perspective on competencies relates to services to *specific populations defined by demographics* such as age (child or adolescent; geriatric) and ethnic identification. Expertise with particular populations may be a result of formal training within any discipline. It may also result from professional experience, or, in the case of minority populations, may be a consequence of personal characteristics of the provider. Selection with regard to this type of proficiency is generally made with little consideration for discipline, on the basis of providers' claims or documentation of expertise.

Specific requirements for composition of a provider network are initially determined by an analysis of the likely service needs of a given beneficiary population. For example, if the benefit plan is union-funded and covers a significant number of retirees, the network should contain providers who are competent to work with an older population. Similarly, if the group includes a significant proportion of Hispanics or particular Asian groups, consideration should be given to bi-lingual professionals or professionals who have experience with these populations and an understanding of the effects of particular cultural factors on psychosocial functioning.

Recruitment and Selection

Those who develop networks generally have two objectives, one immediate and one longer term. The first is to ensure that, by and large, providers initially selected for a particular network are more competent than providers not selected. This requires use of a formal, criteria-based selection process to predict who are the more desirable providers from the system perspective. The second objective is to ensure that the cost-effectiveness of the service system increases over time. Achieving this second objective requires two things: (1) implementation of a formal monitoring process which allows judgments to be made about the adequacy of each provider's performance with respect to explicit criteria for process and outcome of services, and (2) feedback and assistance to providers whose performance is judged to require improvement.

State licensing and even specialty recognition such as board certification provide no guarantee that a professional will be able to provide either the type or the quality of services required by managed systems. Laws and processes governing licensing and credentialing of providers may vary across states, are typically vague, and inadequately address the specific types of services which designated specialists are licensed to provide. In addition, the increase in the numbers of traditional training programs, such as doctoral programs in psychology, as well as non-traditional training and certificate programs (e.g., mental health counselors, chemical dependency specialists, EAP counselors) makes it impossible to determine either the quality of such programs or what competencies the graduates of these programs are likely to possess. In short, managed care companies are left to "fend for themselves" in the tasks of finding, recruiting, and maintaining a high quality provider network.

Finding Candidates for the Network

If the goal is to establish only a very small network confined to a single geographic area, a managed care company might be able to achieve this through an informal process, initially contacting providers known to someone within the company and building on personal referrals from these professionals to enlarge the group of candidates. For networks beyond very small, localized ones, however, formal sources must be consulted to obtain a sufficiently large pool of candidates from each of the required disciplines. These sources are varied, and include lists of licensed professionals obtained from state licensing boards; membership rosters from specialty boards for psychiatry, psychology, and clinical social work; and membership lists from clinical associations such as the National Register of Health Service Providers in Psychology and the American Association of Marriage and Family Therapists.

MINIMUM QUALIFYING CRITERIA. Some companies accept state licensure as the primary qualifying criterion for network membership. Other companies, attempting to maintain a somewhat higher standard, designate additional requirements, typically a minimum number of years of experience and certification by a professional specialty board such as the American Board of Psychiatry and Neurology or the American Board of Professional Psychology.

Practitioners satisfying these minimum criteria are invited to apply for network membership. They generally are asked to submit an application accompanied by proof of licensure and professional liability coverage, and to submit names of two or three professional colleagues who are willing to act as references.

Managed care organizations have a responsibility to exercise "due diligence" in the development of the provider network. This means, among other things, that a company may not rely totally on the self-report of the potential network members to determine that they satisfy the relevant criteria. An independent process for validation of the information provided by candidates must be implemented. The company may rely on a range of resources for validation including direct contact with state licensing boards and professional certifying bodies as well as letters of reference.

Because there is no single national registry or data source maintaining information about health services professionals, the validation process is potentially very time-consuming. As a consequence, several companies have recently been established which provide credentialing services to managed care companies. In addition to validating credentials, these companies will research the litigation history of providers and monitor licensing board disciplinary actions.

Supplementary Criteria Defining "Quality" of Providers

The final step in the process of selecting members for the network is the review of the materials submitted by the candidates and their referees, and validated, at least in part, by the managed care company. Programs vary greatly in the extent to which they utilize additional explicit "quality" criteria at this stage of the selection process. At one extreme are companies which take the position that trying to predict who will be the better providers is a pointless exercise. These companies would typically select network providers on the basis of state licensure; absence of evidence of malpractice judgments, legal or ethical violations; and, possibly, board certification. (This last criterion is regarded as particularly important with regard to the selection of psychiatrists.)

At the other extreme are companies which use seemingly sophisticated criteria for judging the quality of providers. It should be emphasized that these types of selection criteria have little empirical foundation. In general, they tend to reflect the personal biases of the professionals who develop them. They typically encompass two categories: those which relate to professional experiences and those which relate to characteristics and patterns of practice of providers.

CRITERIA RELATED TO EXPERIENCE. Since accountability is an essential element of managed care, some companies give priority for network membership to providers who have experience in what are usually regarded as "accountable" systems. These would include, for example, community mental health centers or other local public mental health programs, Veterans' Administration facilities, and professional training settings within universities, medical schools or other service delivery organizations. Preference is also often given to providers who are a part of group practices, particularly if the practices themselves maintain formal accountability and quality assurance procedures or have demonstrated the capacity to provide particularly cost-effective services.

CHARACTERISTICS AND PATTERNS OF PRACTICE. In addition to accountable providers, managed systems seek professionals whose practices reflect reasonable and cost-effective service provision. Accordingly, information solicited from network candidates often addresses specific aspects of practice. Listed below are examples of indicators which have been used by managed care companies to assist in provider selection.

- *Disorders typically treated:* Providers who seek to limit their practice to disorders such as multiple personality, co-dependency, or adult children of alcoholics—conditions which are seen to reflect treatment "fads" or the diagnoses of which have little empirical support— are viewed more negatively than providers who present themselves either as generalists or as possessing specific proficiencies with respect to particular populations, such as children, older adults, and racial/ethnic minorities.
- *Patterns of outpatient service:* Providers whose typical patterns reflect a focused, time-limited model of service delivery are preferred for network membership over those whose patterns of outpatient care indicate a more long-term, intensive (high frequency) approach.
- *Utilization of inpatient care:* Managed care companies prefer providers who regard inpatient care as an acute treatment alternative appropriate for use only in the most extreme circumstances. They prefer to avoid providers whose patterns of inpatient utilization indicate that they view this modality as applicable for a wider range of habilitative and rehabilitative purposes.
- *Use of alternative outpatient services:* Managed care companies seek

providers who make use of cost-effective group modalities as an alternative, rather than merely as an adjunct to individual treatment, and who refer patients to low cost or free community-based services or self help groups, when appropriate.

- *Utilization of assessment:* Managed care companies look for providers who use formal testing and assessment only when it is necessary for the development of a treatment plan, rather than solely to provide additional diagnostic clarity.
- *Patient load:* Providers who see very large numbers of patients each week may be regarded as having insufficient time to devote to other activities believed to be integral to high quality services such as developing formal treatment plans, writing session notes, and managing referrals.

It should be emphasized that managed care companies which are particularly discriminating with respect to provider selection can expect to have difficulties in establishing a provider network of adequate size and representation. Networks invariably lose members after they have been established. During the selection process the company must, therefore, balance its need to ensure quality "up front" against its more pragmatic need to have sufficient numbers of providers to meet contract demands or satisfy the state regulatory requirements applying to the particular type of service delivery structure.

The Contract

The contract between the provider and the managed care company invariably addresses the financial and administrative (accountability) aspects of the contractual relationship. The latter would include, for example, requirements for submission of treatment plans, discharge summaries and other documentation; the benefit plan requirements for pre-certification, co-payments, etc.; and requirements for cooperation with case managers. The contract may also identify the company's expectations regarding the preferred orientation of treatment and the willingness of the provider to work within the bounds of the benefit plan. This generally means short-to-medium term treatment focused on objective treatment goals, and a rehabilitative approach emphasizing return of the patient to a reasonable pre-morbid, rather than optimal, level of functioning. Benefit plans which guide service provision in managed care companies generally are not intended to support personality restructuring nor to deal with chronic conditions.

Maintaining and Improving Networks

With the exception of those who refuse to comply with the explicit requirements of the managed program or commit some egregious violation of professional norms, providers are usually retained by the network for a period of time during which the company gathers sufficient data to make informed judgments about their adequacy as practitioners in a managed setting. Definitive determinations of provider adequacy can only be made after a thorough evaluation of data relevant to provider performance. The basis of provider monitoring is "profiling": aggregation and reporting of data describing patterns of practice, clinical outcomes, and some administrative aspects of practitioners' performance in the managed care context.

MONITORING CLINICAL PERFORMANCE. Clinical indicators are intended to reflect the quality of the process as well as the outcome of services delivered by the provider. Indicators might relate to:

- outcome of treatment as reflected in standardized assessments, provider ratings of functioning, readmissions, etc.;
- patients' evaluation of the provider and the services received (patient satisfaction survey);
- provider's adherence to empirically based guidelines for process of care;
- case manager's evaluation of the clinical services based on review of treatment reports or consultation with the provider.

Summaries of a provider's performance can be used to identify particular populations or diagnostic groups with which he or she appears to be most effective. Based on such data, managed care companies can become increasingly selective in the process of "matching" providers to patients. The monitoring process, in essence, may effect a gradual movement of managed care providers from the generalist to a specialist category. Consistent with this, there is an evolution within managed care toward "privileging" providers with regard to particular types of diagnoses, problems, or specific clinical procedures. Such an approach is similar to that traditionally used by hospitals with medical staff members in order to improve quality and reduce potential liability due to adverse outcomes.

Monitoring Administrative Indicators. Administrative indicators are intended to reflect how well the provider fulfills his or her responsibilities as an "employee" of the managed care company. Administrative indicators may relate to:

- provider's response to referrals (for example, whether initial visits are scheduled in a timely, appropriate manner);
- ratings of compliance with requirements for submission of treatment reports, discharge summaries, and other documentation;
- case manager's evaluation of quality of his or her interactions with the provider.

The managed care company must balance the clinical performance of the provider against his or her willingness to adhere to those administrative requirements which make the system manageable and accountable. Practitioners who provide cost-effective services but do not comply with administrative requirements present significant challenges for a system attempting to demonstrate accountability to external sanctioners. Different, but equally serious, challenges are presented by the consistently compliant provider who is unable to achieve good clinical outcomes.

The managed care program monitors the providers as a group as well as individually in order to ensure that the network as a whole is competent in the provision of the range of services necessary for the beneficiary populations. Determinations made in review of the system have implications not only for network expansion but also for professional development and continuing education activities.

At the aggregate (network) level, evaluation of practice patterns and clinical outcomes within regions serve the function of a needs analysis—to identify provider training needs within a region and form a basis for the development of appropriate training programs. Examples of topics for training programs which have been undertaken by managed care programs include: short-term treatment for behavioral manifestations of severe personality disorders; the development of measurable treatment goals; and procedures for matching goals and treatment strategies.

Improving Performance by Providing Feedback

Giving providers feedback on the managed care company's evaluation of their performance is a critical task which must be managed appropriately. Through case-specific feedback, the case manager attempts not only to influence the treatment plan but also to acquaint the provider with the principles of appropriate resource utilization. It is, in essence, a process of professional socialization through which providers are introduced to the unique value stance and clinical behaviors required by an accountable system. While these requirements are specified in the provider's contract with the managed care firm, they often take on meaning for the provider only when they are exemplified in context of the case management process.

Feedback may be verbal or written and may address clinical or administrative issues. The clinical issues which are most frequently the subject of comment include: inconsistencies within the treatment plan with respect to diagnosis; lack of specificity of treatment goals; use of unnecessarily intensive treatment strategies; and treatment oriented toward the achievement of optimal functioning rather than the recovery of pre-morbid functioning. Administrative issues include: failure to submit treatment plans or other documents or to submit them on time; provision of frequency, intensity, or type of service not authorized by the company; and exhibiting a generally negative attitude toward the case management process.

A large proportion of providers accept feedback from case managers and modify treatment plans or practice patterns accordingly. In such situations, the relationship between the managed care company and the provider develops in a positive way, the frequency of reviews decreases, and the likely frequency of additional referrals increases. Providers who are less receptive to feedback and fail to develop an appropriate relationship with case managers compromise the managed care company in terms of extra clinical resources, increased per case expenditures, and unacceptable outcomes. Therefore, those who remain resistant or unable to adapt to the needs of the case management process lose referrals or are formally removed from the network.

It is important to recognize that a provider's negative attitudes about the managed care process may be the result of the case manager making unreasonable requests (e.g., requests which can not be justified clinically) or handling the feedback process in an inept or ineffectual manner. Just as there is variation in competence among network providers, so too is there variation among case managers in terms of the attitudes and skills necessary to adequately perform their jobs. The challenge to the managed care company is to train and develop case managers sufficiently skilled to handle the difficult task of giving feedback to providers.

Special Considerations with Institutional Providers

The development and management of a network of institutional providers (facility-based and structured treatment programs) present additional dilemmas for the managed care company. Such entities are more difficult to identify, differentiate, and monitor for quality than are individual practitioners.

Institutional providers include a wide variety of physical settings, including hospitals, residential treatment centers, group homes, therapeutic ranches, and wilderness programs. A variety of programs may be offered within a given setting. These may include acute care, residential rehabilitation, full- and partial-day treatment, social-model chemical dependency rehabilitation, and structured outpatient treatment. Finally, within programs, variations occur with regard to treatment philosophy, intensity and frequency of services offered, types of modalities utilized, and qualifications of the staff providing services. These institutions and programs are often licensed by different agencies within and across states. Hence, identifying and comparing them within a state or nationally can be an exacting task.

The individual differences from program to program also present problems in identification of benchmarks for comparisons. For example, while adolescent treatment programs may have similar physical plants, staff-to-patient ratios, and daily program schedules, they may have very different treatment philosophies and goals for treatment. These latter factors can have a significant impact on length of stay, cost per case, and long term treatment outcomes. It is for this reason that many managed care programs try to limit variation by restricting the types of settings eligible to participate in the network to programs with clearly defined licensure categories. For example, a company may contract with licensed hospital programs, but not with residential treatment centers or group homes.

Once a group of potential institutional providers is identified, the processes of recruitment and selection are similar to those used with individual providers; they are, however, more complex and time consuming. The credentials review process focuses on the licensure and, if relevant, accreditation status, the range of services offered, the components of each program, clinical indicators (such as average length of stay), and litigation history. A representative of the managed care company may conduct a site visit to verify program components, examine staff credentials, and review a sample of medical records. Concurrently, the company negotiates a preferred—usually per diem—rate for that facility or program, and carefully defines the services which will be included within that rate.

Monitoring Institutional Providers

Monitoring the performance of institutional providers presents its own set of challenges for managed care companies. The primary problem is that it is not always possible to assign responsibility for treatment to one individual within an organized care setting. When a patient is in outpatient treatment with an individual provider, that provider is clearly responsible for treatment and, under a managed program, is the appropriate person to be held accountable for compliance with the case management process and for clinical outcomes. In the case of services delivered through institutions or programs, multiple staff are typically involved in directing and providing treatment. In addition to these program staff, there may be one or more independent service providers within the program who are beyond the direct control of the facility. (An example of such a situation would be a psychiatrist on the open medical staff at a hospital where the practitioners' services are billed separately from the facility charges.) The internal case management function which should exist within organized care settings is frequently ineffective, and the representative of the managed care company may end up dealing with utilization review personnel who have little if any contact with the patients in question.

The potential for high costs associated with utilization of institutional providers in terms of patient acuity, dollars spent, and case management resources, necessitates immediate identification of programs that do not satisfy the performance criteria of the managed care company. Consequently, most companies conduct intensive reviews of facilities on a case-by-case basis in addition to monitoring profiles of these programs with regard to routine clinical variables as well as special factors such as adverse outcomes.

Conclusion

The process of network development is still in its infancy, is essentially ad hoc, and lacks any theoretical substratum. At the same time, a significant body of knowledge exists within industrial psychology—a developed technology which could eventually provide an empirical foundation for the complex processes of provider recruitment, selection, monitoring, and retention. The application of this knowledge and its related technologies to network development would not only improve the effectiveness of the selection process, but also render the selection process less vulnerable to legal challenge by providers who are rejected for network membership. Finally, the application of such empirically derived mechanisms could reduce the potential liability to managed care companies for what might be adjudged to be negligent provider selection in the case of malpractice by a network provider (Newman & Bricklin, 1991).

In the final analysis, managed care programs can not alone ensure that their providers possess the skills and attitudes required in the managed care environment. This can only be achieved via collaborative efforts between the industry and professional mental health training programs. It will likely require the passage of a number of training cycles before the effect of such collaboration begins to take effect in the form of provider attitudes and behaviors which are deemed appropriate to the changed world of behavioral health practice.

REFERENCE

Newman, R., & Bricklin, P.M. (1991) Parameters of managed mental health care: Legal, ethical, and professional guidelines. *Professional Psychology: Research and Practice, 22,* 26–35.

Chapter 4

MANAGED CARE AND PROVIDERS. YOU'RE IN BUSINESS!

Nancy E. Lane

Health care costs escalate uncontrollably. Millions uninsured. Outpatient mental health benefits disappearing. Managed care opportunities for providers. Quality assurance and cost containment—better care for less. Precertification and concurrent review—please provide information. Can you reduce the fee, my insurance won't cover this?

Sound familiar? Statements like these currently surround mental health services. Many mental health professionals wonder, How did this chaos develop? How can I survive professionally and economically? How can I even feel good about what I do?

This chapter explores issues in managed mental health care from the vantage point of providers of that care. First, we consider managed care as it has gradually entered the awareness of a 'typical' provider, maybe someone like you. Next, we discuss how managed care has developed in the world outside of the consulting room, and how the future looks. We discuss some ways providers can rethink their roles to become more active and assertive in their dealings with managed care systems. We present practical tips for adjusting clinical practice patterns. And, finally, we consider the possibility that managed care may play a socially useful role while serving to control costs.

What Happened to My Dream?

If you are a typical mental health practitioner, you worked long and hard to get professional training, to develop a professional approach and identity, and to build a practice, whether as a solo practitioner, part of a group, or in a hospital or clinic setting. You may have trained during the boom years of the community mental health movement when funds were plentiful and available mental health services for all seemed an achievable dream. You may have been trained in a very traditional program where you learned highly specialized treatment approaches, perhaps focusing on long-term therapies with the aim of character change. Still others of you may have entered the field through the human potential movements of the 1970s, believing that growth and self-actualization were desirable mental health goals for all people. Many providers looked forward to the day when they could leave their clinic jobs behind and settle into a comfortable independent practice setting where they could provide the services they had devoted themselves to mastering and in which they believed most fervently. The existence of accrediting organizations, licensing, and third-party reimbursements made this possible, at least for a while.

Whatever kind of academic preparation you may possess, and whatever the training context to which you were exposed, it is unlikely that you were taught to consider financial limits or involvement by funding entities in your treatment planning. At most, you may have been taught that fees and their collection are an important part of the clinical "work" between you and your patient. More often, if you were trained in a clinic or hospital setting, fees were the province of the administration, and providers steered clear of this area. If you then went into independent practice, it was often with the longing for a simpler, more private way to do your work—just you and your client, with a few notes and a three-ring binder to keep track of your financial records. Treatment decisions would be made by you and your patient, not according to the demands of managers or supervisors.

But it has not turned out quite that way. In the past ten years, providers have become, at first dimly and now forcibly, aware of the growth of managed care and its profound effects on the way they practice. The first inkling was the establishment of limitations on the number of sessions per year insurers would reimburse. Then the requests for treatment reports started arriving from insurers who were buying utilization and peer review services from outside companies and professional associations. You may have been outraged and refused to cooperate or even sought legal remedies to limit what information you were required to supply. You may have referred patients with what seemed particularly restrictive policies on to other providers. You hoped this trend would blow over as its negative impact on clinical treatment outcomes was exposed. It did not.

The next set of events you may have experienced seemed potentially positive at first. Patients started appearing whose treatment would be covered if you were part of a provider network, or if you were approved as a provider by their insurer or employer. You may have seen this as a new market opportunity. Sign up with a number of these organizations and you could probably have a steady stream of referrals, benefitting from those providers who refused to join the network.

Then the paperwork started and you were asked to fill out lengthy forms about yourself and about your treatment policies. You were asked to report to the referral source every few sessions, in a particular format dictated by them. You had more paperwork to fill out to be paid, and the pay was often at a discounted rate. You were allowed only a limited number of sessions, and for many of the networks you joined, referrals were non-existent. Worst of all, when benefits ended, you were left trying to explain to the patient what had happened.

Meanwhile, Out in the Real World . . .

While providers of mental health care were struggling to comprehend and adapt to the rapidly changing conditions in reimbursement strategies, all organizations involved in funding health care were facing new economic realities. Health care costs, especially those for mental health care, are rising sharply each year. (See Broskowski [1991] for a thoughtful discussion of how and why costs have risen so dramatically.) Employers struggle to provide adequate health benefits for their employees and many of these employers have become self-insured to allow themselves greater flexibility in the types of coverage they extend. Insurers cannot design affordable profitable products that meet consumers' expectations and regulatory mandates. At the same time, the pool of health care providers continues to expand, all of whom are seeking parity and equal access to reimbursement from third-party payors.

It is in this atmosphere that the worlds of health care and business begin to converge. Rodriguez (1989) discusses how management, the uniquely American response to crisis, has been applied, and how it has shaped mental health services delivery and funding. He points to four major areas of activity in cost containment: benefit design and restructuring; alternative reimbursement methods; utilization review and case management; and alternative delivery systems (provider networks, gatekeepers, etc.).

Most providers are probably familiar with certain characteristics of early managed systems, including sharply curtailed numbers of covered sessions and discounting of "usual, customary and reasonable" fees. Less familiar, but rapidly increasing, are requirements for providers to inter- act directly with case management organizations for precertification or concurrent review of treatment. Preferred provider networks, many of which carry both utilization review requirements and limits on payments, are now common. These offer insurers the very attractive possibility of strongly influencing both choice of provider and amount of service covered.

Provider response has ranged from outrage, to professional concern, to active participation. (See Berman et al. [1987] for a discussion of some typical responses.) But the existence and persistence of efforts to manage care and limit costs are constant reminders that business demands and management strategies are now shaping practice in ways unthought of even 15 years ago.

Re-imagining the Future

Providers can begin coping with managed care realities by adding an additional element to their conception of themselves and the work they do. That element is a simple one—that of a business person. You are now in the business of supplying behavioral health services. Marketplace demands and restrictions apply to your work in new ways, but market- place opportunities also appear.

Viewing behavioral health services as a commodity to be bought, sold, marketed, and negotiated requires a shift in thinking. Certainly, the very public marketing of treatments for addictions, eating disorders, prob- lems of adolescence, and depression, among others, indicates a move- ment in thinking toward treatments as units of service available for specific costs. At the same time, however, individual providers are often uncomfortable with marketing themselves directly and few have training or experience to do so.

To begin thinking in a business sense, the mental health professional must ask two critical questions: *Who is my customer?* and *What am I selling?* Previously, in fee-for-service settings, patients presenting themselves for treatment were the customers. Length and type of treatment varied depending on the type of problem presented and the treatment style of the provider. The reimbursing agency did little but process claims and send checks.

Managed care is different. Now, treatment length, style, and even choice of provider may be independent variables controlled by the managed care entity paying for the treatment. Therefore, providers must carefully consider the reality that the patient is no longer the sole customer. A customer is also the managed care system that is responsible for the patient's benefit plan. At the very least, this new third party has an interest in the treatment and must be included in decisions, especially those which have an impact on cost.

Services being purchased under managed care may differ from the products typically offered by traditional mental health professionals: assessment, development of an individualized treatment plan, and delivery of whatever amount of service meets the objectives of that plan. A managed care entity may want to purchase, for example, a particular number of sessions of cognitive therapy to stabilize job performance during a period of major depression. Or it may want providers to work quickly and efficiently rather than allow the concerns of the patient to unfold naturalistically as the therapeutic relationship develops. Finally, it may request that providers assess problems quickly and make referrals outside the managed care system (that is, for care uncompensated by the managed system) for clients who desire growth therapy.

It is uncommon, in our experience, that requests and expectations of managed care organizations are characterized by the level of specificity of the above examples. Their requests are often dismayingly imprecise and sometimes even constitute poor practice. They, as the providers, are new in the managed care business, and they are feeling their way. At the same time they generally present a clear expectation (often combined with a monetary threat) that whatever is to be accomplished be accomplished in a brief period of time and that it be done well. Providers who can articulate what they do, how they do it, why they are doing it in a particular case, and how long it may take to accomplish have an advantage in dealing with managed care organizations. They are more effective sellers of themselves than are providers who view themselves narrowly as, for example, psychoanalysts, behavior therapists, or in any other professional role which suggests that their decisions about treatment are dictated by their identity rather than by the patient's problems.

Certain aspects of conceptualizing behavioral health services as business commodities remain extremely difficult to reconcile from the position of the individual provider. It is disorienting to realize that as a business person you are being asked to develop a professional business and attract users, but then do all you can to ensure they use no more of your service than is absolutely necessary. Some providers respond by expanding their practice to include consultation, education, and other indirect services. For highly specialized providers, this approach may be inappropriate, diluting their effectiveness and making their services less available to those who might benefit.

Providers who inevitably view themselves relatively narrowly as specialists need to think of themselves as elements of larger health care systems which provide a wide range of services. In such systems, specialist providers receive referrals of patients in need of their particular services while case managers coordinate overall treatment and benefits. But there is a subtle shift in power in these systems which providers sense and often resent. Whoever assesses the patient and coordinates the payment, often not the individual provider, plays a vital role in deciding who gets and who performs treatment. Individual providers accustomed to doing assessment and treatment in the private, fee-for-service sector often find this intrusive and demeaning.

So . . . How Can I Respond?

Early responses by providers and professions to managed care were characterized by disbelief and anger. More recently, there is a beginning emphasis on how providers can cope with this new but rapidly growing marketplace environment. (See, for example, Haas & Cummings [1991] and Richardson & Austad [1991].) In this section, we discuss some specific steps you can take if you want to begin repositioning yourself and your practice to respond to and capitalize on managed care.

ADOPT A BROADER VIEW. Begin by trying to broaden your vantage point. Accept that your view of needs for behavioral health services is greatly affected by the small slice of the world you see in your practice. Statistics suggest that most treatment is short-term (often as few as five or eight sessions) and that maximum treatment effects are often obtained by the twenty-sixth session (Garfield, 1986; Howard et al., 1986). There is a residual population of patients who benefit from long-term treatment, and another small number for whom long-term treatment (albeit of varying modalities) appears to be the only alternative (severe character pathology, psychosis, dual-diagnosis, multiple personalities). If you have been in practice a long time, your case load may have a relatively large percentage of these clients. It is important to keep in mind, however, that benefit packages are generally reflective of national utilization statistics (Richardson & Austad, 1991). As such, they may not be hostile in intent, even if they do not take clinical exceptions easily into account.

Look At What You Do. Consider what your actual patterns of practice are. List all the patients who have contacted you for service in the past several years. Note how many came for more than six or eight sessions. If you are a typical provider, it was probably no more than a handful. While most of us provide long-term therapy, we forget how many patients are, in fact, short-term. If you have been in practice a long time, you may have a high percentage of long-term clients who have gradually accumulated on your roster. It is generally these long-term, difficult or complex cases on which we focus and which dominate our memories and cloud the fact that for each patient who settles into long-term treatment there are perhaps ten others who come for only a few visits.

Analyze The Market. Take a broad look at the behavioral health care market and the opportunities that present themselves in your area. Find out who is buying mental health services in your community and what type they are buying.

- Are there still large numbers of people who have traditional fee-for-service insurance?
- Are there one or more large managed care entities which might provide you with a large referral base?
- What are the large employers in your area doing with respect to employee assistance programming?
- Are small employers looking for ways to provide services outside of or in addition to their insurance plans?
- What markets are already adequately or even over-served?
- Have some groups or hospitals cornered the market in certain types of service?

Do A Self-Assessment. After you have analyzed the market, do an honest assessment of what you want to do and what you are *able* to do.

- Is it most important to you that you continue providing a specific service you believe in?
- Are you more interested in expanding the services you offer to include new areas of expertise?

- Is there a particular population, defined geographically, diagnostically, or culturally, that you want to serve?
- Do you want to be in a solo practice or are you comfortable working with a group or in a clinic?

In effect, perform a personal market analysis of what you have to provide, who is interested in buying your services, and who is already in this market. Ask also,

- Can you collaborate or compete?
- Are there areas of unmet needs where your services could be useful?

Once you know what you have to provide and who you might want to provide it to, you can make some decisions about how to position yourself as a provider.

- Are the economic conditions in your community conducive to maintaining a traditional private practice?
- Would you be more comfortable in a clinic setting where an administrative team will be responsible for dealing with marketing and payors?
- Are you interested and willing to take on learning the business of managed care as an individual provider or as part of a small group?

MAKE AN ASSERTIVE APPROACH TO MANAGED CARE. If you decide that managed care is a reasonable professional alternative for you, you are now ready to approach managed care organizations about participation in their programs. A proactive approach may be more useful than waiting to be approached by networks seeking providers or patients suggesting you sign up with certain networks so that their benefits are available. Not all managed care organizations are alike and, by actively investigating them, you may discover ones with which you are compatible and which value your skills.

Managed care organizations are businesses and you will need to evaluate them first from that perspective.

- Is the company financially solvent?
- Do they have a good reputation?
- Do they cover a large enough population to provide you with sufficient referrals to make participation worthwhile?

You will also want to evaluate their business practices. Some specific areas to investigate are discussed by Haas and Cummings (1991). Questions to ask include:

- Who in the system assumes the risk?
- What provisions exist for exceptions to the benefit limits?
- What referral resources are identified for patients whose benefits become exhausted?
- Do they sponsor or subsidize provider training?
- Are they open to provider input concerning their policies?
- How do they communicate with plan participants, both patients and providers?

Once you enter an agreement with a managed care organization, take an active role. Do not be apologetic about what you provide or what you charge. Influence extends both ways in managed care, and providers should insist on having input into areas such as the costs of services and systems of documentation. Ask if your own record keeping system and reports will meet the requirements of the managed care system. Be friendly with the case managers and ask for their help when needed. Expect them to function as professionals and hold them accountable for decisions regarding limitations, exclusions, or extensions of treatment.

Be mindful of the complexities of the patient-therapist-managed care relationship. Insist that the managed care organization take legal and formal responsibility for educating patients about the limitations and exclusions to services provided under their agreement. Ensure that patients know these limitations before beginning treatment. Try not to get drawn into the position of fighting with the managed care organization to provide services they are not contractually obligated to provide. Advocate for patients whose conditions warrant extension or modification of benefits, but have a range of options available in case you are not successful.

You will need also to assess your typical practice patterns and evaluate what you need to change to be more compatible with managed care. For example, you should carefully evaluate your patients' need for longer-term treatment (Lane-Palés, 1989), and develop alternative plans to provide it when indicated. You may have to lower fees so that patients can pay for their own treatment or you may need to refer patients to sliding-scale clinics. At the same time, develop your skills in short-term or intermittent treatment. Do not try to do long-term treatment for a few sessions.

If you have skills and interests in program evaluation, treatment research, or administration, consider selling these services to managed care organizations. Managed care is evolving rapidly and there is need for skilled mental health professionals who can contribute to responsible program development.

Lastly, take time periodically to evaluate how your relationship with the managed care organization is working for you. Change what you can, and leave provider networks you feel you cannot work with. Stay active in professional associations that represent you and your interests. Always be aware that in the changing marketplace you have an opportunity and as well as a responsibility to use your experience and expertise to influence future developments.

Some Final Words

Managed care has been seen as a blessing, a curse, the end of health services as we know them, as well as a bright new opportunity for containing costs while improving quality of services. All of these perspectives are valid to some extent. But for mental health in particular there may be some encouraging aspects which are easily overlooked (Broskowski, 1991).

Behavioral research has been slow to produce large-scale studies of treatments and their effectiveness. As more treatment is delivered in a managed care environment, data will become available about who used services, why, if they were effective, and how much they cost. Such data provide, at last, a basis for programmatic research on the questions of efficacy and cost-effectiveness which have been ignored by the behavioral health professions for so long. This is a welcome possibility, especially if professional behavioral health researchers become involved in such studies.

All practitioners are only too familiar with the fragmented nature of the service delivery system in this country. Outpatient and inpatient care are generally available, but little exists for those in need of partial hospitalization, socialization services, or continued community-based support services for chronic populations. Most providers encounter few of these patients, and insurers have not had to deal with them as a group. Managed care organizations responsible for large groups of enrollees will be in a position to contract for these services from providers ambitious enough to organize them. Lower costs from lower hospitalization rates make such services attractive, and while they are frequently unavailable, many providers believe them to be the treatments of choice for many more patients than those who currently have access to them.

It is difficult to predict what the future holds for individual providers of behavioral health services. But as with any large-scale change in society, the evolution of managed care provides an opportunity and mandate for us all to reassess the value of what we do and work to shape the future to assure we can do it the best we know how. The goal of accountability toward our (multiple) sanctioners may be relatively new, but it will likely not lose its central position in behavioral health service delivery. There are many ways to be responsive to such a goal, and each is a challenge to the new professionalism managed care will extract from service providers.

REFERENCES

Berman, W.H., Kisch, J., DeLeon, P., Cummings, N., Binder, J., & Hefele, T. (1987). The future of psychotherapy in the age of diminishing resources. *Psychotherapy in Private Practice, 5,* 105–118.

Broskowski, A. (1991). Current mental health care environments: why managed care is necessary. *Professional Psychology, 22,* 6–14.

Garfield, S. (1986). Research on client variables in psychotherapy. In S. Garfield & A. Bergin (Eds.), *Handbook of Psychotherapy and Behavior Change.* New York: Wiley, 213–256.

Haas, L. & Cummings, N. (1991). Managed outpatient mental health plans: clinical, ethical, and practical guidelines for participation. *Professional Psychology, 22,* 45–51.

Howard, K., Kopta, S., Krause, M., & Orlinsky, D. (1986). The dose-effect relationship in psychotherapy. *American Psychologist, 41,* 159–164.

Lane-Palés, N. (1989). Explicit clinical assessment for appropriate longer-term therapy. *Psychotherapy in Private Practice, 7,* 3–12.

Richardson, L. & Austad, C. (1991). Realities of mental health practice in managed-care settings. *Professional Psychology, 22,* 52–59.

Rodriguez, A. (1989). Evolutions in utilization and quality management. *General Hospital Psychiatry, 11,* 256–263.

Chapter 5

BEHAVIORAL HEALTH CASE REVIEW: UTILIZATION REVIEW OR CASE MANAGEMENT? ONE COMPANY'S VIEW

Bettie Reinhardt and Gary L. Shepherd

This chapter provides a description of the process of behavioral health case management as it is conducted by one specialty case management company. The chapter is organized around two primary themes: (1) the role of the case manager and how he or she actually makes the case management process work; and (2) what the case management company can legally and practically do to affect patient treatment. In an effort to vivify the case management process for the reader, we include examples of actual cases encountered by the authors in their years of managing cases.

The Goal of Case Management

Our primary goal as case managers for behavioral health services is to increase the probability that the patient receives the appropriate mental health or chemical dependency treatment at the time that it is needed. To accomplish this, we attempt to influence the patient's treatment through active participation in its planning and careful monitoring of the treatment process.

A secondary goal which guides our work is to ensure that the patient receives high quality services. Quality of health services is a complex concept. It includes, at a minimum, consideration of treatment outcome or effectiveness, treatment process, service costs, service availability, and service acceptability to the patient. In context of a managed system, the definition of quality becomes even more complex. It includes consideration of all the aspects mentioned, in addition to effectiveness of the case management process and acceptability of the process to both the service provider and the patient. Under a managed system, then, high quality services yield desired outcomes, are delivered via modalities and other processes which are accepted by professional and regulatory bodies, and are provided at the lowest possible cost, in sites and at times which make them accessible to the patient. In addition, the services are perceived by the patient and his or her family as being acceptable, and by the provider as being appropriate to the patient's needs. Finally, the process through which the case manager works with the provider and the patient intrudes minimally on the patient's sense of entitlement and on the provider's sense of professional autonomy.

Obviously, a service can not maximally satisfy every aspect of quality in every case. Each requirement (e.g., cost, acceptability) is, in fact, a constraint, and each constraint acts to shape the services in a particular way. For instance, a particular benefit plan may establish cost as a primary constraint by limiting dollar amount, number of visits or days, or type of service to be covered. A critical question for the case manager, then, is "How can the desired outcome be reached given the limitations of the benefit plan?" While cost may be the primary constraint, our primary concern as case managers is treatment outcome.

Effect of Case Management on Cost

There is some evidence that case management can, and does, result in lower behavioral health care costs by encouraging the use of cost-effective, alternative service types and shorter term treatment. If a single, complex case (the type most likely be selected for case management) is viewed over its entire history, service costs will likely be less if the care has been managed. At the same time, if a case is viewed from a short term perspective, management may actually increase costs. For example, a case manager may identify the need for a more highly trained or more costly service provider (e.g., adding a physician to the treatment team for medication consultation), for additional services (e.g., recommending a complete psychoeducational assessment for a child whose problems include school adjustment), for more intensive services (e.g., increasing the number of sessions during a period of exceptional stress), or even for a more restrictive setting (e.g., suggesting residential treatment for an adolescent whose family is unable to support outpatient treatment due to deterioration of the family system). Such short-term cost increases should result, ultimately, in cost savings in the longer term.

The basic facts about case management—its objectives and priorities and their consequent effect on costs—must be understood by all parties who are affected, directly or indirectly, by the process. The employer or payer who believes case management will inevitably prevent the occurrence of expensive cases may well be dismayed when such a case presents. The case management company, therefore, should ensure during the contracting process that the payer has realistic expectations for what case management can and can not accomplish over the short and long term.

Beneficiaries must understand before they seek treatment that case management is an integral part of the service process and that the objective of the case manager is to be an advocate and resource for the patient. The care giver, similarly, must understand that providing services under a managed system brings with it an array of formal responsibilities, and that the case manager is most usefully seen as a professional colleague and resource person.

What Case Management Companies Can Do

Formal case management differs in one very important respect from the management of services traditionally performed by service providers themselves. That is, while the service provider *determines what type and how much of a service to deliver* to the patient, the case management company *determines which, if any, services should actually be paid for* by the insurance or health plan. In the former situation, the provider is practicing his or her profession, whether it be medicine, psychology, or social work. The case management company, however, may not legally engage in behavioral health service delivery. Hence, the case manager may not mandate a treatment plan, and he or she may not require the patient to be discharged from a treatment setting, even if review determines an absence of medical or psychological necessity. Finally, the case manager may not require an individual service provider to admit the patient to a particular treatment setting or provide a particular type of service, even if a review has determined such a service to be medically indicated.

On the other hand, the provider has no authority to decide which service should be an insurance or health plan benefit (except in the rare situation where he or she has a contract with the payer to do so). It is the authority of the case management company to make the benefit determination which gives the principal weight to its decision. Review and case management companies regularly disclaim their responsibility for treatment determinations and reaffirm their role in determining treatment benefits.

A TAXONOMY OF REVIEW AND CASE MANAGEMENT

The case management process as it is most commonly practiced has evolved out of less comprehensive processes of service monitoring classified as utilization review (UR). UR is the practice of judging services against predetermined criteria or norms for clinical appropriateness, medical or psychological necessity, and length of stay (LOS). Case management carries with it some level of responsibility for patient care. In particular, the case manager assumes the responsibility for identifying and recommending for the patient those services which he or she believes will most effectively and efficiently return the patient to the expected level of functioning. This responsibility remains with the case manager as long as the mental health services are deemed to be required. Although the case management system does indeed commonly utilize the traditional UR strategies, its overall focus is by no means restricted to such strategies.

Current models embody the evolution of the UR process. It is often difficult accurately to discriminate the approaches of review companies, some of which refer to themselves as UR companies, and those which claim to be case management operations. While a key variable is the extent of control, or responsiblity assumed by the reviewer in each kind of operation, the centrality of the reviewer role is not invariably the factor which best discriminates between the two approaches. Thus, for illustrative purposes we have conceptualized UR and case management activities on a continuum (see Figure 1).

It is important to note that Figure 1 does not provide a definitive taxonomy of review and management models. Rather it is intended to exemplify the types of relevant variables and direction of variations which are frequently observed in UR and case management organizations. The key is intended to provide a better understanding of the way characteristics of the process change as one moves from UR to case management.

The point labelled "1" in Figure 1 represents utilization review in its earliest and simplest form. Under this model, the primary activity is retrospective monitoring and reporting of utilization and practice patterns. A left-to-right movement along the continuum brings models utilizing concurrent and prospective, as well as retrospective, review procedures.

Figure 1

Range of Utilization Management Activities

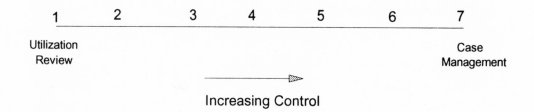

| 1 | 2 | 3 | 4 | 5 | 6 | 7 |

Utilization
Review

Case
Management

Increasing Control

Key to Figure

1
Retrospective process
Determination of norms
May compare expected LOS to actual
May develop provider profiles
May enter feedback loop with provider

3
Concurrent process
Determine appropriateness of admission
Identify expected LOS
Compare what is occurring to expected
Encourage providers to work toward expected
May make payment recommendations

5
Concurrent/prospective process
Make treatment recommendations prior to admission
Make determination of treatment appropriateness
Make recommendations regarding treatment
    appropriateness
Participate in discharge planning
Recommendations often include a range of options
Recommendations are made to payer and reported to
    providers

7
Concurrent/prospective process
Participate in patient evaluation
Participate in treatment planning
Direct contact with patient, family, provider
Recommendations relate specifically to facility and
    professional provider
Recommendations made to provider as well as payer
Recommendations carry weight of benefit determination

The position represented by point "4" could reflect the intensity and type of UR typically conducted. Under this model, for example, the necessity of a hospital admission which has just occurred, or is imminent, is determined by comparison of characteristics of the clinical situation with explicit criteria. An admission determined to be necessary is approved for a specified number of days (typically between 3 and 7). To receive reimbursement for more than this number of days, the provider-in-charge must request an extension and supply clinical justification for the continued stay.

The model represented by point "5" would probably include some case management functions. Under such a model, the reviewer may, in addition to approving a specified number of days or sessions to be reimbursed, suggest an alternative level or type of service which he or she believes might be more appropriate for the patient. These suggestions tend to be rather general in nature and the reviewer has no authority to enforce them. Under such a model, also, the UR reviewer may employ peer reviewers (i.e., peers of the providers) as consultants who may communicate directly with the provider and discuss alternate treatment strategies. (All review programs have some access to peer or consultant reviewers. Traditionally, their role under UR is to endorse a denial of benefits.)

What distinguishes case management (which would be represented by points 6 and 7) from the UR models preceding it on the continuum is the fact that under the former process the case manager assumes responsibility for identifying the appropriate services and providers. Indeed, the case manager's recommendations are quite specific, and these recommendations carry with them the formal weight of a benefit determination (i.e., payment for services). The following example provides an illustration of the critical difference between UR and case management.

Example 1: The Deteriorating Family System

Seven year old Jimmy Smith, experiencing hallucinations and agitation, was brought to the hospital by his mother, a single parent. Mrs. Smith reported that he had been having a consistent problem with sleeplessness. Jimmy was admitted on an emergency basis to the children's unit where immediate evaluation was undertaken by a multi-disciplinary team including a child psychiatrist, a child psychologist, and a social worker. A hospital representative called the review company to request authorization of benefits for the admission and for several continued stay days.

The psychiatric nurse conducting the review determined that the severity of

Jimmy's condition warranted treatment at the level requested by the hospital. She approved the admission and, guided by LOS criteria, approved a specific number of days. She told the hospital representative that she would call back periodically during this time period for status reports on the child, and that for additional days to be approved the attending professional would need to call her at least 24 hours prior to the expiration of the current approval with a progress report and a revised treatment plan to justify the additional days.

It should be noted that, while case management companies prefer high cost services such as inpatient care to be preauthorized, they acknowledge that certain conditions might require emergency admission before the review company can be contacted. In such cases, they require that the treatment facility contact them within 24 hours of the patient's admission. If such an admission is determined by the review company to be unnecessary, the facility itself is liable for the cost of the services provided during that 24 hours.

The review nurse in Example 1 made, in effect, a UR determination. Using written criteria and standards for "medical necessity" to guide her, she determined that Jimmy's condition was serious enough to justify admission. Using additional standards for length of stay, she approved a specific number of days of care. She expected to obtain additional information from the hospital and the physician during the hospitalization to determine whether evidence for medical necessity continued to be present, whether services appeared appropriate, and whether discharge planning was occurring as it should. When she received the first report on Jimmy's progress, she received additional information which made the case appear significantly more complicated.

> Jimmy became frantic to see his mother, an alcohol-dependent woman with only a brief history of sobriety. Mrs. Smith's two other children, John and Lisa, were demonstrating similar preoccupation with receiving their mother's, and anyone else's, attention, and were exhibiting severe behavior problems. John, in particular, seemed depressed and the psychiatrist suggested admitting John to the hospital. Mrs. Smith described her family's life as chaotic and said she had no idea what she should be doing for or with her children.

More than utilization review was needed at this point. All four members of this family were in need of help—immediately and probably for the foreseeable future. The family's contact with mental health professionals had so far been limited to the inpatient context. Since the inpatient setting is appropriate for acute needs only, not for longer-term treatment, the hospital would not be able to provide all of the services needed by this family. In addition, once the inpatient treatment was completed (and after the hospital's discharge planning responsibilities had been fulfilled) the family would be left with no identifiable resource person to help them through the maze of available community-based services.

The review nurse decided that case management was called for, primarily because of the complexity of the family's needs, but secondarily because without the ongoing support of case management the family situation was likely drastically to deteriorate. Someone needed to take the longer-term view, to work with the mother to establish some long-term goals for the family, and to identify and help the family obtain access to the range of services needed for it to reach a reasonable level of functioning and stability.

This family required a range of psychosocial services, not only the traditional treatment (i.e., "therapy") services. In fact, additional assessment of the family situation, of the mother's ability to cope with the children, and her ability to control her substance abuse problem indicated that the three siblings would be better served by a temporary alternative living situation.

> The case manager encouraged the hospital social worker to provide extra family sessions immediately. This additional support to the family enabled John to remain on an outpatient basis while his apparent depression was evaluated. He was found to require medication and was admitted to the hospital long enough to establish the appropriate dosage. Upon discharge from the hospital, John was transferred to a residential treatment center (RTC) and Jimmy soon joined him there. The RTC was recommended by the case manager because she was familiar with its program and believed it would be good for both boys. Furthermore, the RTC maintained day treatment services and had arrangements with several foster families who provided temporary living arrangements for children who were attending the center's day treatment program. Hence, with the help of the RTC, the case manager arranged for a foster family to provide temporary shelter to the three Smith children. The children could be together, the boys could "transition out" of residential treatment by way of day treatment, and Mrs. Smith could have a needed respite.
>
> Mrs. Smith required not only parent effectiveness training and support, but ongoing support for her chemical dependence rehabilitation. Some of the services most useful to her were available in the community in the form of 12-step groups and parenting classes at the community college.

Case management does not create miracles. The Smith family, however, are functioning out of the hospital setting and there are no indications that their functioning will deteriorate.

Identifying Cases Requiring Management

In view of the demonstrated importance of early interventions in mental health, it is critical for case management organizations to have the capability of identifying at an early treatment stage cases which might benefit from case management intervention. While some cases will be recognized by case managers on the basis of their experience and professional judgment, case management organizations typically look to the literature as well as to the experience of the organization to develop formal written criteria for identifying such cases.

The criteria generally include reference to variables which have been shown to be associated with high cost cases, whether for reasons of clinical presentation, provider patterns of practice, or patient compliance. Table 1 provides a sample list of criteria. In Example 1, above, the Smith family satisfied criteria relating to the areas of life functioning affected, the ability of the family to support treatment, and the number of family members experiencing problems.

We now present an example in which the reasons for case management related both to the clinical issues and to the payer's fear of legal consequences if the requests of the provider and the patient were not granted.

Example 2: The Insistent Patient and Provider

Marsha had been in outpatient treatment with the same therapist for several years. Since her health plan reimbursed for individual outpatient therapy without requiring review, neither Marsha nor the therapist had any direct contact with review personnel during the years of treatment. At one point, Marsha and her therapist agreed that treatment had been going on too long without the desired results and that a change in treatment setting might break what they saw as an impasse. In particular, the therapist decided, and Marsha agreed, that several months of inpatient treatment might allow her to break down Marsha's defenses in a safe setting.

As required by the benefit plan, the therapist requested prior authorization for the inpatient admission from the case management organization. At the time of the request Marsha was still functioning well on the job and had just been promoted, although she was experiencing increasing anxiety at work. While she had significant dysfunctions in the social and family areas of her life, the problems were not of a severity which would require inpatient services.

Table 1

Foci of Criteria for Selecting Mental Health Cases to be Managed

---

Patient Variables

- Severe dysfunction in more than one area of life (i.e., work, school, family, peer relations, legal, social, self care)
- Multiple problems or needs
- Chronic mental illness
- Recurrent mental illness
- Severe character pathology
- Previous mental health or chemical dependency inpatient treatment

Family and Social Support Variables

- Multiple family members requiring significant mental health or chemical dependence treatment
- Low to minimal social supports
- Low to minimal family support
- Pathological family system

Legal and Situational Variables

- Patient or family history of appeals
- Patient or family history of litigation
- Provider history of appeals
- Provider history of litigation
- Provider history of non-cooperation with managed care or utilization review
- Provider history of non-compliance with professional guidelines

Treatment and Provider Variables

- Provider use of unusual treatment modalities
- Change of diagnosis after admission
- Report of continued presence of suicidal or homicidal ideation after one week of hospitalization
- Continued stay beyond target LOS date for reported diagnosis and severity

---

The UR reviewer did not approve reimbursement for the inpatient admission, but because Marsha and her therapist were persistent in their attempts to obtain authorization, the reviewer (guided by the criteria) recommended that a case manager be assigned to the case.

Formal assessment revealed that Marsha had significant problems in every area of life functioning except work. She exhibited rather severe character pathology and was involved in a dysfunctional family system. The case manager obtained a consultant's evaluation of the outpatient therapy and it was determined that the therapeutic relationship was basically useful, and further that the patient had the capacity to achieve the desired outcome.

At this point, the case manager consulted with the therapist and the patient in an effort to set up an alternative treatment program that recognized both the patient's needs and her strengths (principally her job performance), and which satisfied the case manager's need to keep Marsha out of the very costly and unnecessarily restrictive acute care setting.

> The case manager had knowledge of a local hospital which provided the type of intensive services which Marsha and her therapist preferred, but outside of a traditional inpatient program. The program included therapeutic and peer support groups, most of which met in the evening, combined with what was referred to as "night treatment." Marsha was to spend the evening attending the groups, sleep at the hospital, and leave early the next morning for work. This allowed Marsha to have intensive treatment and to receive the peer and other support necessary to make use of the therapy, while continuing to be productive and successful in her job. She was able to achieve the transition from the hospital program to outpatient groups that, along with individual therapy, provided the treatment components that individual therapy alone was not able to provide. As a result, Marsha progressed out of her "treatment rut."

In Marsha's case, the indications for case management were two-fold. First, she had significant dysfunctions in more than one life area. Second, she and her therapist were insistent on obtaining more intensive services and, in the judgment of the reviewer, were likely to initiate legal action if the requested admission was not approved.

Did the management of Marsha's care save the health plan money? Clearly not in the short-run, since inpatient treatment had already been denied. But, by shortening the course of individual therapy, by reducing its frequency in favor of outpatient groups, and by intervening in ways which were likely to prevent the cycle of self-endangerment and hospitalization that many patients with severe characterological problems confront, the case management system probably saved the health plan money in the longer term.

It is certain that case management was associated with cost savings for the employer, from both long- and short-term perspectives. The increased cost for the more intensive services was more than offset by the fact that Marsha continued in her job and, by doing so, saved the company the cost of hiring and training Marsha's replacement. Marsha's overall functioning was improved and her job functioning was preserved and enhanced.

A Closer Look at the Case Manager's Role

The case manager's professional role involves at least five separate functions:

- Identification at an early treatment stage of cases which will benefit from case management
- Assessment of patient's needs, strengths, and available support systems as well as potentially appropriate community resources and providers
- Identification and assistance to the patient in accessing of the most effective and efficient services
- In cooperation with service providers, provision of guidance to the patient and family during the course of treatment
- Communication with and coordination of activities of clinicians, treatment programs, payers, patient, and family.

To do these things well, the case manager must be well versed in information about general treatment issues and possess comprehensive information about the services available to the beneficiaries of the managed care system. In particular, the case manager must be familiar with information concerning:

- Efficacy of the range of treatments for particular problems, as reported in the professional literature
- Effectiveness of facilities, programs, and clinicians, as reflected in his or her experience working with them and in the pattern of practice profiles generated by the managed care program
- Availability and quality of self-help and other psychoeducational programs in the community.

The case manager must also have well developed communication and clinical skills. We assert that the behavioral health case manager should be a clinical specialist—psychiatric nurse, social worker, psychologist, or psychiatrist—with significant experience in both inpatient and outpatient settings.

While well developed competencies are essential if the case manager is adequately to perform the clinical aspects of his or her job, such skills are equally important when communicating with service providers and programs. Because the case manager adopts the role of active service broker and advisor on treatment options, he or she needs to establish as quickly as possible manifest competence in the eyes of the professionals who are participants in the management process.

What the case manager does not do is just as important as what he or she does. The case manager should not convey the attitude that he or she, by virtue of the job title, has a greater knowledge of what is best for the patient than the clinicians working with the patient. The case manager's role is different from the role of the service provider, not lesser and not greater. He or she is a member of the treatment team, a resource person, a coordinator, and a service broker.

Most behavioral health professionals have some experience on multidisciplinary teams. The difference is that, under managed systems, the teams have a de facto member. When a case manager actually attends team meetings at a facility, it is generally easier for providers to view this third party representative as a team member. Physical presence is often not possible, however, due to cost considerations and geographical limitations. The case manager, then, is manifest as a voice on the phone, and it may be easier under these circumstances for the service provider to perceive the reviewer as a personification of the insurance company rather than as a mental health professional colleague.

In our experience doing review primarily by telephone, one of the most difficult aspects of managing a case is establishing a relationship with the provider such that the provider is receptive to the case management process. This is facilitated enormously if the case manager possesses highly developed communication skills. Above all, however, the case manager must demonstrate competence. Everything that he or she says must reflect expertise in the treatment of the type of patient whose care is being managed, and knowledge about intervention options and available community resources.

The corollary is that the case manager should not attempt to manage a service about which he or she has little expertise or knowledge. For example, if a case manager has no experience with substance dependence treatment programs, he or she should not be given the responsibility for a "dual diagnosis" patient. To do so is counterproductive and serves only to reinforce providers' prevailing negative attitudes about case management.

We believe that personality characteristics and maturity are the two factors which best separate effective case managers from merely adequate or ineffective ones. The case manager must frequently, under non-conducive circumstances, be able to get providers and patients to "hold hands and sing" even when they are not sure they like the song. To achieve this, the case manager must convey a personal warmth, a respectful attitude, and a positive outlook that engenders both trust and a willingness on the part of providers and patients to cooperate. Even the most professional and strategic approach by the case manager does not, of course, guarantee success. This being so, the case manager must often maintain a positive and professional attitude in the face of what may be biting hostility and attempts by providers to attack and demean.

Professional Status Issues

The majority of case managers are psychiatric nurses or social workers. This is because there are more of them than there are other (doctoral level) mental health professionals, and they cost less to employ.

There are times when the front-line case manager needs to involve a psychologist or psychiatrist. This may be necessary when the case requires more expertise than the nurse or social worker possesses. It also occurs frequently, however, in the situation which may be called the "battle of the degrees". What follows is a not atypical example.

Example 3: A Matter of Status

An attending psychiatrist described a recently admitted patient to the nurse case manager as being clinically depressed with constant ruminations about his "wasted life". He reported also that the patient had been compliant with an antidepressant regimen prior to admission, but the drug had not prevented the development of vegetative signs or the ruminations.

Since the medication had not been changed since the admission to the hospital, the nurse asked the psychiatrist if he was considering a change. She also asked him if he had considered trying one of the newer antidepressants that had been shown to reduce obsessive thought processes. In response to this inquiry, the outraged provider focused on the temerity of the nurse who, he perceived, was "telling him how to practice medicine".

When the case manager was unable to refocus the psychiatrist on the patient's treatment, she withdrew and asked one of her company's psychiatrist consultants to speak with the attending. The consultant was quite direct (and directive) with the psychiatrist—indeed, much more so than the nurse had been. He made very specific suggestions regarding types of antidepressants and dosages, recommendations which were totally consistent with the recommendations made earlier by the case manager.

In contrast to his behavior with the nurse, the provider listened politely to the consultant. He and the consultant spoke in a collegial manner about their respective experience with depressed patients, and there were no accusations about the consultant interfering in the treatment of the patient.

In this example, it is clear that the message was less important than the messenger. The reader should not assume, however, that the doctoral level consultants themselves never meet with hostility from providers. It probably occurs less frequently than with masters level case managers, but tends more frequently to include denigration and personal attacks by the service provider. A common accusation from service providers is that the consultant does not care about patients, and is concerned solely with effecting savings for the insurance company.

So, Why Do We Do It?

On balance, case management is a rewarding job. It provides the support and motivation for maintaining knowledge about current therapies and services and for sharing that knowledge with people who can use it to provide more effective treatment services. It offers opportunities for sharing experiences with other professionals with an equivalent commitment to high quality care. It provides the opportunity to become acquainted with a far greater variety of behavioral health professionals and service settings than would occur in a traditional clinical practice. It provides the opportunity directly to assist patients and families as they attempt to find their way through the maze of services which pass as the health system in the U.S. Finally, it is at the very heart of the growing climate of accountability in health services delivery.

We conclude this chapter with an example which highlights the potential of case management for direct intervention with patients.

Example 4: Direct Intervention with the Patient

Tony, a prospective patient, called the UR nurse to obtain authorization to enter an inpatient alcohol treatment program. While Tony's description of the extent of his drinking indicated that he had a significant problem, he did not satisfy the criteria for either inpatient detoxification or inpatient rehabilitation. Hence, he was told that, while an inpatient program would not be paid for, an outpatient program would be. In response to the denial of reimbursement for inpatient services, he insisted that there was nothing else for him to do but to continue to drink. He was referred to case management.

The referral was for two reasons. The first was that the UR nurse believed Tony had a legitimate need for treatment, but, left to his own devices, he would probably not become involved in any treatment program. The second reason was that Tony appeared to lack an understanding about the range of treatment alternatives and their relative appropriateness for different types of patients.

> The case manager talked to Tony and learned that what he wanted was for people—his wife, his boss—to stop "hassling" him about his drinking. He did not believe he had a drinking problem and he was not ready to commit to sobriety. The case manager determined that, because of the apparent lack of motivation for treatment, a formal rehabilitation program of any type was not appropriate but that the Alcoholics Anonymous (AA) program and some one-to-one counseling to support the referral to AA might be helpful. This strategy would allow Tony to be seen as complying with the wishes of his wife and boss (hence, it would be seen by him as an acceptable alternative). At the same time, the case manager believed that the experiences with AA and the counselor might help him develop motivation for treatment.
>
> The case manager talked to Tony about the referral to the AA program (she gave him a telephone number and the name of a person to contact), and she referred him to a counselor. She stated specific expectations that Tony would need to meet before payment would be forthcoming (that Tony attend at least one AA group and that he keep all appointments with the counselor) and she set dates to follow up with him by telephone. A letter was sent to Tony confirming the expectations and providing information about 12-step groups available to Tony's family.

The case manager will monitor Tony's ability to use this level of intervention and his need for, and ability to profit from, other interventions as time goes on. If Tony does decide that more intensive services are appropriate for him, the case manager will be prepared with information about appropriate alternatives and about other community resources which may be accessed by Tony's family.

PART III
LEGAL AND REGULATORY INFLUENCES:
HELP OR HINDRANCE?

PART III: INTRODUCTORY NOTE

Governments, both federal and state, have had significant impact on the form and substance of health services in the U.S. They achieve this by exerting influence both as makers of law and regulation and as purchasers of services. In the former capacity, they provide enabling legislation or financial assistance, in the form of tax incentives, loans, or subsidies, to encourage the development of service systems which complement current health policy. As purchasers they offer substantial markets, such as Medicare, to providers and service systems which are able to satisfy requirements related to factors such as service cost, format, organisation, or quality.

The federal government has been particularly successful in stimulating the development of models of managed care through both these roles. In Chapter 6, DeLeon, Bulatao, and VandenBos describe two major federal government initiatives. The first is the 20-year program of legislation and financial subsidies aimed at encouraging the development and implementation of health maintenance organizations (HMO). The HMO is critical to the discussions in this book since it provided the original model for managed care. Indeed, for many years it was the *only* managed health services delivery system which existed. HMOs were originally created and have been in operation since the early 20th century, but their growth was limited until the mid-1970s when the federal government first made an explicit commitment to the model and provided legislation and subsidies to encourage its development.

The second initiative discussed in Chapter 6 is that undertaken by the Department of Defense (DoD), Civilian Health and Medical Program of the Uniformed Services (CHAMPUS) as a purchaser of services for seven million CHAMPUS beneficiaries. The DoD exercised its significant buying power and its authority to regulate the shape of health structures—sometimes overriding state laws—in order to encourage the development of a new type of managed service delivery system.

Another area of legislation pertinent to health services delivery relates to state licensing and policing of health care providers. State governments have been consistently unable to ensure the competence and appropriate behaviors of professionals through such regulatory means. In Chapter 7, Dörken discusses two types of legislative efforts by the state of California: (1) law and regulation pertaining to the licensing of health professionals and intended to protect the public; and (2) legislation intended to stimulate the use of professional peer review for dealing with incompetence and raising the quality of health services. With regard to both legislative efforts, the primary goals of the legislation have not been realized in California—nor, indeed, in other states under similar legislation. As a consequence, the managed care industry has, for pragmatic reasons, intervened in areas previously believed to be the domain of state regulators by developing its own mechanisms to serve the original intent of such laws.

Chapter 6

FEDERAL GOVERNMENT INITIATIVES IN MANAGED HEALTH CARE

Patrick H. DeLeon, Elizabeth Q. Bulatao, and Gary R. VandenBos

In its twin roles as purchaser of health services and facilitator of the development of innovative health care programs, the federal government has had a significant impact on the development of managed care programs. In this chapter, two programmatic initiatives are discussed from the perspective of their impact on the evolution of managed behavioral health care: health maintenance organization (HMO) development, and the implementation of managed care strategies within the Civilian Health and Medical Program of the Uniformed Services. HMOs are given particular significance in the chapter since, until 1980, the two terms, "HMO" and "managed care," essentially referred to the same structures and mechanisms. It was only during the 1980s that managed health care truly came to capture broader and more varied health services delivery and reimbursement mechanisms.

What is an HMO?

An HMO is a health services organization that enters a contract to provide a predetermined range of medical and other services to a designated population for a fixed premium, usually referred to as a "capitation rate" (Flinn, McMahon, & Collins, 1987; Koch, 1988). It has two primary characteristics which give it the incentive and the potential to provide higher quality services at lower cost than the traditional fee-for-service system. The first is that the HMO assumes a financial risk. If the cost of services provided exceeds the amount of the premiums (the "prepayment" amount) the extra cost constitutes a loss to the HMO. This feature provides a disincentive to the over servicing which is typical of fee-for-service plans. The second characteristic is that services are provided by a defined group of professionals who are responsible for the total health status of the enrollees. Such an arrangement gives the HMO the control necessary to achieve the most cost-effective allocation of resources within the service system. In their attempts to maximize the cost-effectiveness of their services, HMOs generally focus on prevention and early intervention.

The Government's Commitment to Health Maintenance

President Nixon's 1971 and 1972 Health Messages to Congress were, for all practical purposes, what brought the concept of managed health care into modern health policy. The President's expressed goal under his National Health Strategy was to "build a true 'health system'—and not a 'sickness' system alone. We should work to maintain health and not merely to restore it" (Nixon, 1971).

This notion of a health care system emphasizing health maintenance, disease prevention, and wellness, along with the concept of the HMO, were adopted by the Nixon administration, and the concepts were expressed legislatively in the Health Maintenance Organization Act (HMO Act) of 1973 (PL 93-222). This philosophy and the model were also adopted by all subsequent U.S. Administrations. For example, the support of the Bush Administration was made quite clear by Health and Human Services (HHS) Secretary Sullivan during 1991 Senate Appropriations Committee hearings when he stated that managed care was "the best means of assuring quality service and appropriate care for Medicare and Medicaid beneficiaries" (Sullivan, 1990).

Federal Legislation on Health Maintenance Organizations

This section reviews the development of federal support for HMOs. It focuses on the federal government in the two major roles which it has traditionally played within the health care arena: (a) that of establishing or facilitating the development of innovative service delivery models, and (b) that of providing care to federal beneficiaries, either directly or through various contract agreements, as a purchaser of care.

The Government as Facilitator: HMO Legislation

Variations of HMOs—all sharing the two fundamental features of prepayment and group practice—have been in existence since early in the twentieth century. While the two most notable programs are probably the Ross Loos Medical Group, organized in 1929, and Kaiser

Permanente Health Plan, fully recognized in 1945, precursors to modern HMOs were organized as early as 1906 (Flinn, McMahon, & Collins, 1987). There was quite limited growth in HMOs until the early 1970s, however, when the federal government made an explicit commitment to the advancement of this model.

In its role as facilitator, the federal government provided significant funding and legislated other incentives for the development of new health maintenance organizations. The HMO Act of 1973 provided loans and subsidies in the amount of $325 million over the first five years of the initial ten-year plan ("HMO law includes," 1974) to encourage the creation and expansion of HMOs. The law also required employers with more than 25 employees to offer the option of joining an HMO as an alternative to its existing health plan, if a federally qualified HMO was available in its area, and if that organization asked to be included among the options offered to employees.

The Act created a certification process, known as "federal qualification", through which HMOs could become eligible for the subsidies. To be qualified, HMOs were required to meet certain financial and organization standards and to provide a comprehensive set of eight basic services, including outpatient mental health care and crisis intervention services, and treatment and referral services for alcoholism and chemical dependency. Other basic benefits included consultation and referral services; emergency health services; home health services; and preventive health services such as voluntary family planning, infertility services, and preventive dental care for children.

In addition to providing loans and subsidies to HMOs, the 1973 act also allowed profit-making corporations to become a part of this health program. For-profit organizations had not been associated with the HMO movement up to that time. The law also opened the door to the "medical care foundation", the forerunner of the independent practice association, or IPA (Bennett, 1988).

In enacting the HMO Act of 1973, the federal government aspired to address what was perceived by Congress to be the increasing difficulty experienced by millions of Americans in attempting to obtain prompt, appropriate health services. Noting the escalating costs of health care even back in the early 1970s, the Senate Committee with jurisdiction expressed the hope that the development of HMOs throughout the country would provide consumers with a greater opportunity to choose the manner in which they would receive and pay for health care—to increase the degree of pluralism in a highly homogeneous industry. Emphasizing how effective HMOs had been, the Committee further maintained that their competitive pressure had a salutary effect upon all health insurance and medical practice. Although it was perhaps not as clearly articulated at the time, those involved in developing this legislation also hoped thereby to significantly modify the "usual and customary" practice of medicine, by awarding greater attention and economic resources to the evolving knowledge base concerning "health promotion and disease prevention" activities (Sen. Rpt. No. 93-129, pp. 7–8).

Amendments made to HMO legislation in 1976 (PL 94-460) and 1978 (PL 95-559) had the general effect of liberalizing the requirements of federal qualification for such status. These new rules provided greater support for the development of HMOs through increased funding and through such strategies as reducing the range of required benefits, increasing the length of time before an HMO is required to offer open enrollment, and exempting HMOs from certain certification-of-need restrictions (Haglund & Dowling, 1988). HMOs were given authority to contract for professional services with individual health professionals or groups of health professionals who did not themselves qualify as medical groups or IPAs, provided that the dollar amount contracted for did not exceed a specified value. Similarly, HMOs were authorized, for the first time since the program's inception, to utilize the clinical expertise of "other health care personnel", which would include nurse practitioners and clinical psychologists.

The Government as Purchaser: Medicare and HMOs

In its role as a purchaser of health care, the federal government created a new market for HMO plans under the Tax Equity and Fiscal Responsibility Act of 1982 (TEFRA, PL 97-248). Under the new rules, Medicare beneficiaries could, for the first time, be routinely enrolled in federally qualified HMOs and in similar entities called competitive medical plans.

TEFRA made major changes in the way the Medicare program reimbursed HMOs. The legislation provided that the financial arrangements between Medicare and the HMO under a risk contract would be comparable to those prevailing in the private sector. The HMO would receive a fixed monthly capitation payment for each enrolled beneficiary and would be fully at risk for the provision of all Medicare-covered services, including physician services, hospital inpatient services, outpatient services, skilled nursing facility, and home health care.

The TEFRA rules took effect when the Secretary of HHS certified to Congress in June 1985 that a satisfactory method for establishing premium rates had been developed. But prior to that time, from 1982 through 1984, the Secretary had entered into demonstration contracts with 26 HMO organizations, using a general statutory authority to waive legal requirements in order to test program improvements. By the end of 1984, 117,588 beneficiaries were enrolled in these experiments. As of September 1987, 1.1 million of the 22.5 million Medicare recipients were enrolled in HMOs, and in 1990, estimates were that the numbers had increased to 1.8 million of the 33.2 million Medicare beneficiaries (Adler, 1990).

Subsequent amendments have been aimed at strengthening the monitoring of quality of care within HMOs and at eliminating alleged abuses in the areas of marketing, enrollment, disenrollment and financial management. To deal with the "conflict of interest" that arises when an HMO provider deciding on patient care has an economic incentive to limit treatment, a provision was included in the Omnibus Budget Reconciliation Act of 1986 (PL 99-509) ensuring that, effective April 1, 1990 (subsequently delayed to April 1, 1991), an HMO or competitive medical plan would be subject to civil penalties if it makes a payment to a physician as an inducement to reduce or limit services to beneficiaries enrolled under a contract with Medicare or Medicaid.

CHAMPUS and Managed Care: The Government as Purchaser

This section reviews the actions of the federal government in its role as a purchaser of care under the Civilian Health and Medical Program of the Uniformed Services (CHAMPUS). This Department of Defense (DoD) program is responsible for providing health care for approximately seven million dependents of active duty personnel, retirees, and the dependents of retirees and deceased military personnel. The general operational policy has been that, where possible, DoD directly provides necessary care through its own facilities and utilizes CHAMPUS, a traditional fee-for-service plan, to purchase care from the private sector only when appropriate services are not available through DoD facilities. The Department's Fiscal Year 1991 budget request for health care was $13 billion, of which $2.9 billion was targeted for CHAMPUS.

CHAMPUS Efforts to Managed Care

Since 1977, DoD, through the CHAMPUS program, has been in the forefront of developing aggressive mental health utilization and "peer review" mechanisms which are, in fact, a form of managed care (Penner, 1993). Their efforts, however, were not expanded to medical-surgical services until the mid-1980s.

Between 1981 and 1984 total CHAMPUS costs increased 7.3 percent faster than private sector health costs. Indeed, by the late 1980s, DoD was experiencing annual unbudgeted cost overruns due to CHAMPUS of $300 to $400 million, resulting in a doubling of CHAMPUS costs over a five-year period of time. In response to these escalating CHAMPUS expenditures, and cognizant of the fact that 26.3 percent of Federal Employee Health Benefit Program beneficiaries were by that time enrolled in HMO plans, DoD decided to significantly expand its previously limited experiments with a "managed care approach", announcing the CHAMPUS Reform Initiative (CRI) in June 1986 (Mayer, 1986).

The policy notions underlying the CRI program were as follows: DoD would be using its nationwide buying power to improve and expand services. The contractor was to be financially at risk, assuming financial responsibility for virtually all health care services provided under CHAMPUS. The contractor would be expected to develop a network of health care professionals and institutions who were willing to provide quality care at reduced rates. Priority would be given to providing preventive care, and careful clinical management would be instituted to offset potential financial incentives for providers to utilize unnecessary inpatient treatment or excessive diagnostic testing and clinical interventions.

There were to be three enrollment options available to CHAMPUS beneficiaries, including the right to remain with their current fee-for-service CHAMPUS coverage. DoD's original plan was to award three such contracts, covering the entire U.S. The Department expected to phase in CRI over a three-year period, starting with a one-year demonstration, to be followed, if successful, by nationwide implementation. However, during the actual "bid process" only one potential contractor emerged. Accordingly, beginning August 1, 1988, CRI services were offered on a more limited basis, in nine catchment areas covering the states of California and Hawaii.

The experiences with CRI in California and Hawaii point to significant potential of the model for both reducing costs and satisfying the needs of consumers. These two states account for approximately 865,000 CHAMPUS beneficiaries, representing 14 percent of the total CHAMPUS beneficiary population. DoD indicated that CRI enrollment reached over 55,000 individuals by October 1989, which was substantially more than expected for the first 15 months of activity. Between 1988 and 1989, the total costs involved increased by 4.5 percent; but in comparison, nationwide, excluding California and Hawaii, CHAMPUS costs had increased 17 percent. At the same time, DoD reports, that of the CRI beneficiaries who had formed an opinion about the medical care they received, 97 percent claimed to be satisfied, and a majority reported they would recommend the program to a friend (U.S. Department of Defense, December 1989).

Despite the apparent successes of CRI, the program has been subject to complaints, particularly from service providers, about problems such as delays in reimbursement, confusing and contradictory guidelines, increased paperwork and perceived unreasonable limitations on mental health benefits (Buie, 1988; Fisher, 1986). As of this writing, Congress has delayed any expansion of CRI.

Additional Efforts Aimed at Mental Health Expenditures

From the beginning, CRI had an especially dramatic impact on the delivery of mental health care in California and Hawaii. The biggest decrease was found for professional and outpatient mental health services. Excluding adjustment, the costs for these services decreased by 34 percent. It is significant that this occurred in the presence of the apparently high level of consumer satisfaction noted above.

Despite the successes of CRI and the continuation of the CHAMPUS mental health utilization review programs (Penner, 1993) total mental health costs still more than doubled between 1986 and 1989, from $303 million to $633 million. In 1989, mental health care represented about 25 percent of the total CHAMPUS program costs, as compared with approximately 11 percent in the private sector, with Blue Cross/Blue Shield reporting only four percent.

CHAMPUS reliance upon inpatient care has been especially severe, with the most recent data available from DoD indicating that inpatient care accounted for approximately 80 percent of the entire mental health account. Accordingly, during its deliberations on the FY '91 Appropriations bill for DoD, the Senate, and subsequently the House-Senate conferees, included a provision which expressly prohibited mental health professionals from admitting patients to clinical facilities in which they have an economic interest. Although the implementing regulations have not yet taken effect, relevant data from the state of Hawaii suggest that within a year, the number of inpatient admissions may be reduced by up to 40 percent. The conferees also included a general provision which allowed DoD to modify CHAMPUS deductibles and to place restrictions on availability of non-emergency care if beneficiaries decline enrollment where managed care programs exist.

Status of Mental Health Within Federal HMO Legislation

Notwithstanding the absence of any legislative restrictions or prohibitions, mental health care is a relatively new addition in health maintenance organizations. Despite their commitment to comprehensive care, with few exceptions the prototype HMOs of the 1940s and 1950s did not include benefits or treatment for mental illness (Bennett, 1988). In the 1960s, in response to the influence of large purchaser groups, including the Federal Employees Health Benefits Program and unions, HMOs started including mental health care on an optional (rider) basis. New HMO plans that emerged in the 1960s, such as the Harvard Community Health Plan, included substantial mental health care as a basic benefit (Bennett, 1988). In general, however, through the early 1970s, there were still numerous questions about the effectiveness of psychotherapy and other mental health treatment, and most mental health providers were not recognized in the majority of reimbursement plans, managed or otherwise, public or private.

The 1973 HMO Act failed to give a solid legislative mandate regarding the provision of mental health services in HMOs. The federal qualification requirement for emergency and outpatient crisis mental health intervention services, one of the basic benefits, consisted of up to 20 visits per year. Alcohol and substance abuse service provision was also mandated. The initial legislation was somewhat imprecise concerning the nature and extent of such coverage, however, and administrative interpretation of this legislation has allowed considerable latitude in services provided (Cheifetz & Salloway, 1984). This has emerged as an increasingly large problem over time, particularly among IPAs.

The potential for over-utilization, inappropriate utilization, and runaway costs related to mental health care were early concerns among managers of comprehensive managed health care plans. However, an evaluation of Kaiser-Permanente's experience with psychotherapy and medical utilization showed that the inclusion of mental health benefits within a comprehensive health care plan did not threaten to bankrupt the health care financing system (Cummings & VandenBos, 1981). Early in Kaiser-Permanente's experience of providing capitated health care, the organization discovered the value of providing mental health services to prevent over-utilization of medical facilities by otherwise healthy persons who were having physical symptoms which were psychological in origin. This is now referred to as the "medical offset effect" of the provision of mental health services (Mumford, Schlesinger, Glass, Patrick, & Cuerdon, 1984).

The typical HMO utilized a single entry point, or "gatekeeper" (usually a primary care physician), to mental health services. This model has generally been viewed as a significant barrier to the appropriate utilization of these services in HMOs (Shadle & Christianson, 1988). The two criticisms of the model are that the physician may have a financial incentive to deny access and that the typical physician gatekeeper does not have the sophistication about mental health services to make appropriate referrals. In contrast, Kaiser-Permanente provided "service on demand" by utilizing multiple entry points for gaining access. Their objectives were to ensure access among patients who otherwise might over-utilize medical services and to treat those patients using structured, cost-effective strategies. The Kaiser-Permanente plan demonstrated that mental health utilization rates were predictable and that mental health is insurable. Utilization rates rose to a predictable level and remained stable thereafter.

Despite the Kaiser experience and the fact that the outcome has been well-publicized over the years, the majority of HMOs still do not provide patients with unrestricted access or multiple entry points to mental health care.

Just three years after the initial HMO legislation was passed, the legislative requirements relating to mental health services in HMOs were somewhat weakened as a result of the HMO amendments of 1976, which sought to reduce the competitive disadvantage of HMOs relative to traditional insurance programs and health delivery systems. Amendments to the HMO Act have appeared periodically from 1975 until the present. The majority of them have not had major implications for mental health services within HMOs. Although the mental health field had actively lobbied for expanded and explicitly articulated HMO mental health services, the 1978 HMO amendments essentially ignored mental health issues.

Growth of HMOs and Managed Care Systems

Federal legislation has been critical to HMO growth. In 1970, prior to the initial HMO legislation, 33 of these organizations covered three million persons (1.5 percent of the U.S. population). By 1980, 236 HMOs covered 9.1 million persons (4 percent of the population). By 1983, 280 HMOs covered 12 million persons (5 percent of the population). By 1987, the number of HMOs reached 707 but it then began to fall, down to 623 at the end of 1989. Further declines up to 1994 are currently projected. Industry sources explain the declines as due primarily to general economic conditions resulting in bankruptcies and industry consolidation. Indeed, enrollments are not declining; 5 to 6 percent annual growth was maintained in the late 1980s. In 1990, an estimated 37 million persons were enrolled, and by 1994 the number is projected to reach 53 million (Marion Merrel Dow, Inc., 1990).

The significance of federal assistance to this growth is manifest. In the eight years following the 1973 legislation, the federal government provided $145 million in grants and $219 million in loans to support 115 HMOs (National Industry Council for HMO Development, n.d.). Early projections of HMO growth under President Nixon were too optimistic, but later projections fell short of actual growth (DeLeon, Uyeda, & Welch, 1985). A ten-year plan developed under President Carter projected 450 HMOs with 20 million enrolled by 1988 (DeLeon, VandenBos & Kraut, 1984). The actual figures that year were 659 HMOs nationwide, serving about 33.7 million individuals.

The "classic" model of an HMO has been a group practice, or staff, system. By the late 1970s, criticisms of such closed panel models by both consumers and providers led to the development of loosely contracted IPA models of managed health care. In the late 1970s and early 1980s, the majority of the new HMOs utilized the IPA model, which tended to be physician-dominated.

Problems and Current Concerns

While some studies of HMOs suggest fairly good availability of mental health services in HMOs, the quality of such care has been questioned, the creation of active barriers to access has been noted, and the exclusion of access to non-physician providers, such as psychologists and social workers, has been legally challenged (Buie, 1990).

In the early years of the HMO movement, much of the interest seemed to center on the delivery of accessible, high-quality health care to a fairly large population at an affordable cost. A number of observers have commented on a lack of concentration among HMOs since 1980 on their role as vehicles for improving quality of, and access to, health care. The rapid development and proliferation of HMO delivery systems have generated considerable debate and criticism from health care professionals and the public. Most recently, common concerns have included that HMOs are used primarily as means of controlling costs, as a source of investment opportunities, and as a means of restructuring the medical care system (Luft, 1987; Shulman, 1988). In Florida, for example, numerous complaints prompted the GAO to conduct an investigation of the new Medicare HMOs. The GAO found these HMOs to be under-regulated by the federal government. They also found that those regulations that did exist were not being enforced—to the detriment of Medicare patients (General Accounting Office, 1988).

The primary areas of concern with regard to the provision of mental health services within managed care settings involve three central issues: access, quality, and consumer awareness.

ACCESS. It is argued that the delivery of mental health care as well as other services to consumers in managed care systems may be inappropriately restricted because of the physician gatekeeping process. The use of such referral controls becomes more questionable when the gatekeeper has a financial incentive to limit access to care. It should be emphasized that federal statutes do not dictate to HMOs *how* services are to be provided—the traditional physician gatekeeper model reflects "common practice," rather than a government imposed standard.

QUALITY. The quality and appropriateness of the mental health services provided through managed care systems are often considered inadequate, especially by private sector providers. The minimal amount of psychotherapy provided and the use of physician gatekeepers who are typically untrained in the mental health area are often cited as evidence of the lack of industry concern about quality and appropriateness of care. Further, there is continuing debate on the definition, value, and effectiveness of the "short-term [not to exceed 20 visits], outpatient evaluation and crisis intervention mental health services" stipulated in the 1973

HMO law. Analysts point out that because the law is not precise concerning the nature or extent of mandated mental health services, administrative interpretation of this legislation encourages latitude in eligibility criteria for outpatient mental health services and in the range of such services provided. Thus, the extent and costs of mental health services provided are actually dictated less by law and regulation than by ways in which HMOs variously interpret and implement such regulatory principles (Cheifetz & Salloway, 1984). Despite the increasing evidence of the effectiveness of time-limited and brief psychotherapy, some mental health professionals still argue that HMOs provide a few hours of "crisis intervention" in the name of "psychotherapy," and that such services are inadequate to the needs of many potential service users.

CONSUMER AWARENESS. Consumers are often not provided comprehensive information about the operation of the managed care plan and the financial arrangements offered by the managed care entities. This has been referred to as "misleading advertising". These entities tend to emphasize only the favorable comparisons between their services and those of traditional health insurance (i.e., that office visits and routine physicals are free, and that there are no deductibles or co-insurance requirements).

The concern with cost-containment and the debate on whether HMOs actually reduce health care costs have prompted various studies comparing service and cost variables between HMOs and traditional-fee-for-service health care arrangements (see, for example, Carlisle, Siu et al., 1992). In general, the conclusion has been that HMOs provide a level of quality no lower than, and possibly in advance of, that associated with other delivery systems. The claim for industry-wide cost reductions as a result of HMO-type management of services has yet to be unambiguously demonstrated.

Impact of Federal HMO Legislation on Clinical Practice

The nature of mental health clinical practice in HMOs has been shaped, albeit indirectly, by many factors, including HMO legislation, market forces, and innovations in the field. Moreover, the clinical experiences of mental health practitioners working in HMO settings have had a broader impact on the general field of mental health as well as on all of health care. This is largely because of the exposure of such providers to an array of other health care professionals with whom they would not otherwise have contact, a range of clinical problems not customarily seen in specialty mental health settings, and a broader range of patient populations.

At the time that mental health services were initially included in the federal HMO legislation, routinely available care could be categorized into a few quite specific areas: crisis intervention, psychotherapy, inpatient psychiatric hospitalization, inpatient detoxification programs, and — less frequently — psychological testing. In reality, the majority of services provided were either short-term inpatient custodial care or outpatient psychotherapy that was either psychodynamic or eclectic in orientation. This situation has changed, however, as some HMOs have made serious attempts comprehensively to address the range of behavioral health needs of their beneficiary populations.

Because of the intentional time and resource constraints maintained in HMOs, as well as the broad array of patient problems confronted by the behavioral specialists in HMOs, mental health providers in such settings have been at the forefront of development of structured, short-term treatment approaches to an array of psychological and behavioral issues. They have also been among the leaders in the development of areas of behavioral medicine and health psychology. In addition, because the basic goal of the HMO is to provide comprehensive health care, all mental health practitioners in HMOs must assume broader roles as health professionals who can contribute meaningfully to the evaluation and management of health problems beyond their traditional roles as psychotherapists. Indeed, multiple roles are common in HMOs, and include administration, organizational consultation, patient advocacy, clinical consultation, teaching, supervision, and research.

There have been criticisms that mental health professionals working in HMOs have "abandoned" traditional psychotherapy approaches or some traditional mental health patient populations. It is probably more reasonable to view the effects of HMOs on mental health providers in a positive light, as significantly contributing to the expansion of both the armamentarium of the mental health provider and the nature and types of problems which they may appropriately address.

Implications for Mental Health Professionals

Relatively few mental health professionals understand the nuances of functionally integrated health delivery systems, and the majority of providers have little or no practical experience working within the various managed care models. Further, relatively few understand that organized systems of care provide the most appropriate vehicles for instituting the "health promotion and disease prevention" activities that every U.S. surgeon general has advocated since *Healthy People* was released by President Jimmy Carter in 1979.

As the nation's health delivery systems are forced to become more cost-conscious, the traditional approaches to mental health education and training which ignore cost as a factor in developing treatment strategies become increasingly untenable. The ways in which professionals work will be influenced by factors in addition to the narrowly defined mental health needs of the individual patient. They will be influenced by the broader conceptualization of behavioral health, which is most appropriately dealt with from a multi-disciplinary perspective, and by service system imperatives to implement cost-effective treatment strategies.

The expansion of health care delivery by HMOs has been a *de facto* national health policy for the United States for over 18 years. This national policy has had significant impact: one out of every seven Americans receive their health care through managed health care systems. All indications are that the federal HMO initiative will continue for a long time. As psychiatrists, psychologists, and social workers become increasingly involved in managed care programs, their respective disciplines will have to contend increasingly with the substantial challenges of a complex and changing system of financing and organization. Nonetheless, absent the strategic focus of successive federal administrations on HMOs and managed care variants, the nature and scope of the challenges with which professions will have to contend would be very different indeed, and the world of practice significantly less enhanced.

Conclusion

Since the mid-1970s, the federal government has been actively encouraging the development of HMOs and other forms of "managed care", both in its role as a purchaser of health services for federal beneficiaries, and in its efforts aimed at stimulating innovative health delivery models. The policy debates surrounding the movement consistently feature the issues of access, cost-containment, and comprehensiveness of services. Over the years, there has been growing awareness of the importance of providing high-quality behavioral health care through managed care systems, paralleling the growth of the behavioral health field in general. However, to fully capitalize upon its potential, the provider community must recognize that managed care systems, such as HMOs, provide a highly appropriate vehicle for instituting the growing interdisciplinary knowledge base inherent in the health promotion and disease prevention field.

Finally, the current debate on issues such as access, quality, consumer awareness, and provider acceptance is full of contention and acrimony. We see this as healthy. That this debate possesses creative and informed elements owes much to the assertive and long term role played by the federal government in HMO and managed care development.

Note. This chapter contains a condensation of information presented in two articles, "Managed Mental Health Care: A History of the Federal Policy Initiative" by Patrick H. DeLeon, Gary R. VandenBos, and Elizabeth Q. Bulatao which appeared in the February 1991 issue of *Professional Psychology*, and "Psychotherapy in HMO Settings: Integrating Federal Policy with Clinical Practice" by Patrick H. DeLeon and Gary R. VandenBos in Austad, C.S. and Berman, W.H. (Eds.), *Psychotherapy in Managed Health Care: The Optimal Use of Time and Resources*, American Psychological Association, 1991.

REFERENCES

Adler, T. (1990, April). HMO fever: Bush budget spotlights managed health care. *APA Monitor, 21*, 17–18.

Bennett, M.J. (1988). The greening of the HMO: Implications for prepaid psychiatry. *American Journal of Psychiatry, 145*, 1544–1549.

Buie, J. (1988, January). CHAMPUS project draws mixed reviews. *APA Monitor, 19*, p. 18.

Buie, J. (1990, March). HMO's quality of care challenged by lawsuits. *APA Monitor, 21*, p. 13.

Carlisle, D.M., Siu, A.L., Keeler, E.B. et al. (1992). HMO vs. fee-for-service care of older persons with acute myocardial infarction. *American Journal of Public Health, 82*, 1627–1630.

Cheifetz, D.I. & Salloway, J.C. (1984). Mental health services in health maintenance organizations: Implications for psychology. *Professional Psychology: Research and Practice, 15*, 152–164.

Cummings, N.A. & VandenBos, G.R. (1981). The twenty years Kaiser-Permanente experience with psychotherapy and medical utilization: Implications for national health policy and national health insurance. *Health Policy Quarterly, 1*, 159–175.

DeLeon, P.H., Uyeda, M.K., & Welch, B.L. (1985). Psychotherapy and HMOs: New partnership or new adversary: *American Psychologist, 40*, 1122–1124.

DeLeon, P.H., VandenBos, G.R., & Kraut, A.G. (1984). Federal legislation recognizing psychology. *American Psychologist, 39,* 933–946.

Fisher, K. (1986, December). Continued role seen in CHAMPUS. *APA Monitor, 17,* p. 29.

Flinn, D.E., McMahon, T.C., & Collins, M.F. (1987). Health maintenance organizations and their implications for psychiatry. *Hospital and Community Psychiatry, 87,* 255–263.

General Accounting Office. (1988). *Medicare physician incentive payments by prepaid health plans could lower quality of care.* (GAO/HRD-89-29). Washington, D.C.: U.S. Government Printing Office.

Haglund, C.L. & Dowling, W.L. (1988). The hospital. In S.J. Williams & P.R. Torrens (Eds.), *Introduction to Health Services.* New York: John Wiley & Sons, 160–211.

HMO law includes mental health services as basic benefit (1974). *Hospital and Community Psychiatry, 25,* 257–261.

Jones, K.R. & Vischi, T.R. (1979). Impact of alcohol, drug abuse, and mental health treatment on medical care utilization. *Medical Care, 17*(12), 1–82.

Koch, A. (1988). Financing health services. In S.J. Williams & P.R. Torrens (Eds.), *Introduction to Health Services.* New York: John Wiley & Sons, 335–370.

Luft, H.S. (1987). *Health Maintenance Organizations: Dimensions of Performance.* New Brunswick, NJ: Transaction Books.

Marion Merrel Dow Inc. (1990). *Marion managed care digest — HMO edition.* Kansas City, MO: Author

Mayer, W. (1986, June). Letter to members of Congress.

Mumford, E., Schlesinger, H.J., Glass, G.V., Patrick C., & Cuerdon, T. (1984). A new look at evidence about reduced cost of medical utilization following mental health treatment. *American Journal of Psychiatry, 141,* 1145–1158.

National Industry Council for HMO Development. (n.d.). *The Health Maintenance Organization Industry Ten Year Report, 1973-1983: "A History of Achievement, a Future with Promise."* Washington, D.C.: Author.

Nixon, R. (1971). Special message to the Congress proposing a National Health Strategy. *Public papers of the presidents of the United States* (pp. 170–186). Washington, D.C.: U.S. Government Printing Office.

Penner, N.R. (1994). The road from peer review to managed care: Historical perspective. In S.A. Shueman, W.G. Troy, & S.L. Mayhugh (Eds.), *Managed Behavioral Health Care: An Industry Perspective.* Springfield, Illinois: Charles C Thomas, 29–44.

Shadle, M. & Christianson, J.D. (1988). Organization of mental health care delivery in HMOs. *Administration in Mental Health, 15,* 201–225.

Shulman, M.E. (1988). Cost containment in clinical psychology: Critique of Biodyne and the HMO. *Professional Psychology: Research and Practice, 19,* 298–307.

Sullivan, L. (1990). Testimony before the Defense Subcommittee of the Senate Appropriations Committee, March 1990. Unpublished.

U.S. Department of Defense. (1989, December). *Report to Congress on the CHAMPUS Reform Initiative Demonstration Project.* U.S. Senate Report No. 93-129.

Chapter 7

MANAGED CARE INTERVENES WHERE STATE REGULATION FAILS

Herbert Dörken

A considerable body of empirical evidence speaks to the efficacy of behavioral health services. Indeed, without such evidence and consensus on the appropriate use of specific intervention techniques, care can be controlled but it can not be managed. In effect, by managing services, managed care companies have come, of necessity, to assume responsibilities previously held to be the exclusive domain of professional training programs and state licensing boards. While regulatory entities and training programs generally strive to ensure that providers are competent and that they engage in appropriate professional behaviors, both approaches suffer from significant inadequacies.

Managed care companies necessarily depend heavily upon expert professional judgments to continue to improve the quality of their clinical decisions. Traditionally, such judgments have been implemented as part of a peer review process, in which the work of professionals was reviewed—retrospectively—by members of the same professional group and, sometimes, of the same subspecialty. In the context of managed care, peer review is more broadly defined as the application of expert clinical judgments by professionals about the work of other professionals. Although for many years peer review was the only generally accepted procedure for making judgments about professional services, it has been both under-utilized and inappropriately used, despite legislative initiatives to encourage its use as an accountability mechanism.

It should be noted that the development and implementation of a peer decision-making process will not alone ensure that a managed care system is effective. To truly "manage" services, organizations require not only a process which encompasses professional review of individual clinical episodes, but also formal accountability structures, such as guidelines for selecting cases for review and for providing feedback to providers.

The appropriate use of expert professional decision-making, then, is a necessary but not sufficient condition for effectively managing the process of care.

A major thesis of this chapter is that the evolution of managed care in its many forms has contributed significantly to the furtherance of two related goals previously thought to be appropriately advanced solely by legislative means: (1) ensuring competence in professional practice and (2) the maintenance of reasonable standards in practice by the use of peer review.

Efficacy: Prerequisite to Managing Care

If the outcome of treatment is not reasonably predictable, if no one form of treatment can be shown to be more successful than others for a given condition, if no particular focus of training can be shown to yield more competent practitioners or practitioners who are better able to serve patients with special needs, and if there is no consensus among practitioners as to what constitutes effective treatment, there can be no rational guidelines for quality assurance nor, indeed, any informed rationale for service provision. Absent these fundamental elements, it can not be claimed that care can be managed—although, of course, it can be limited.

From the perspective of a managed behavioral health care organization, the critical question is: *Do we have sufficient knowledge and skills to achieve predictable outcomes?* If the answer is negative, efforts to manage care are essentially futile.

Despite the absence of a definitive "yes" to the question of efficacy, there is a growing body of empirical research demonstrating that psychotherapy can be effective. The comprehensive review of Jones and Vischi (1979), for example, showed that there was significant empirical evidence of the effectiveness of psychotherapy. In their meta-analysis of psychotherapy outcome studies, Smith and Glass (1977) reached the same conclusion. Further, evidence exists that the appropriate use of behavioral health services can reduce total health care costs among high utilizers of medical services (Follette & Cummings, 1967), among patients recovering from acute illnesses and surgery (Mumford, Schlesinger & Glass, 1984; Devine & Cook, 1983; and Gruen, 1975), and among the chronically ill (Schlesinger, Mumford, Glass, Patrick, & Sharfstein, 1983).

It is interesting to contrast evidence about behavioral health with what is known about general medical-surgical services. In 1978, the federal Office of Technology Assessment reviewed the efficacy and safety of medical technologies and concluded that "only 10 to 20 percent of all ... medical procedures have been shown by controlled tests to be beneficial. . . . " This conclusion contrasts with statistics related to the effectiveness of mental health treatment. Smith and Glass (1977) concluded from their review of a large number of outcome studies that the average client treated with some form of psychotherapy, the primary treatment strategy used in mental health, "is better off than 83% of those untreated with respect to alleviation of fear and anxiety. The improvement in self-esteem is nearly as large." It appears, then, that the empirical rationale for service provision may be no less compelling in the case of mental health services than for medical care.

In addition to the growing body of evidence that psychotherapeutic treatments are effective, there is increasing acceptance of the importance of identifying specific interventions to target specific complaints. For example, a succession of investigators have demonstrated the efficacious application of behavioral and physio-behavioral techniques to chronic pain as well as a variety of physical problems, including Raynaud's disorder, hypertension, migraine headache, muscle retraining and incontinence (Fordyce, 1988). With regard to mental health problems, many anxiety conditions appear particularly responsive to specific behavioral interventions, and depression has been shown to be effectively treated with cognitive behavioral techniques. The "one size fits all" approach in which a generic procedure is used regardless of presenting problem, and which most directly serves the convenience of the provider, can no longer be defended—if, indeed, it ever could.

Two characteristics of the behavioral health field, then, have critical implications for the management of care. The first is that behavioral health services are, or more accurately can be, effective for a range of behavioral and physical problems. Many of these intervention strategies have an acceptable scientific base and there is consensus about their appropriate use. These facts provide the basis for care management.

The second characteristic is the increasing specialization in behavioral health practice. Indeed, the increase in the need for specialization far outstrips the capacity of existing education and training structures to appropriately prepare professionals for practice, and governments to regulate to ensure competence in practice. Managed care firms, therefore, need to have access to a range of specialist and other expert professional advice to ensure that equitable and effective mechanisms are developed and implemented and appropriate judgments made in the process of managing services. They also need to be involved in continuing professional development of practitioners.

The New Practice Environment

With the proportion of the U.S. Gross National Product consumed by health care approaching 14%, public concerns with regard to health services are shifting from provider-patient relationship issues to issues of access and affordability. A partial response to this dynamic is increasing entrepreneurism and cost competition in health care. Health services for a growing number of Americans are being provided by large health care corporations. The cottage industry of independent practice is increasingly threatened by this growing competition and the shrinking of the portion of the market which offers traditional "freedom of choice" of provider. Increasing numbers of providers are contracting with managed care organizations at discounted rates, and even forming their own delivery systems and marketing behavioral health services to employers. Since government is the major purchaser of health care services, further regulation based on a "prudent buyer" philosophy can be anticipated.

In this environment the competitive focus has turned from price alone to "value for money" in health services. The primary objective of managed care companies is to develop systems which, in essence, will improve the cost-effectiveness of the services which they sell. To do this, these systems must improve their capacity to evaluate the generic competence of potential network providers and to ensure their adequate clinical performance in the new context of managed care. It was held, traditionally, that these imperatives were the responsibilities of professional training programs and, subsequently, of licensing boards. The pace of change in health care has far outstripped the capacity and—some would say, the willingness—of such institutions to uphold the tenets of accountability and to protect the public.

Mechanisms for Public Accountability

Traditionally, the fundamental bases for ensuring public accountability have been as follows: (1) the established national and regional standards for professional training and specialty accreditation; (2) state licensing laws which define minimum qualifications and scope of practice by profession and contain some provisions relating to appropriate professional behaviors; and (3) a formal process of continuing education or professional development to ensure that practitioners remain current with developments in their field. Collectively, these mechanisms have a modest potential to protect the public by ensuring that persons who hold themselves out to the public as practitioners have received an identifiable core of education and demonstrably possess a core of knowledge and a minimal level of competence in the application of such knowledge. In fact, the above mechanisms were intended to provide protection against only the most flagrant violations of professional guidelines.

The objectives of licensing laws are both to define the boundaries of professional competence and manage incompetence (Overholser & Fine, 1990). In the interest of the latter objective, all such laws include mechanisms for the ongoing monitoring of professional behaviors and for acting on public complaints. To the extent that they do this they play a vital role as an external accountability control mechanism (Wiens & Dörken, 1986). But such laws have been demonstrated to be inadequate in substance and in function.

Licensing of Professionals

Each state in the U.S. has developed a range of law and regulation which may expand or constrain the scope of practice, or place specific requirements upon licensees as a condition of practice. Scope of practice generally embraces the entire range of services that members of those professions might provide. In other words, licensing is usually "generic." The presumption is, of course, that no one member of a licensed profession can reasonably have or sustain competence in such a panoply of activities, and it is, again presumably, left to post-licensing credentialing programs to ensure specialty competence.

The range of services defined for emergent professions, such as psychologists and nurse practitioners, commonly designated as "limited license" or "allied" practitioners, are typically more narrowly defined than scope of practice set in statute for established professionals, such as physicians (psychiatrists). There are many pressures on states to maintain constraints upon the emergent professions. Generally these pressures derive from competing professional groups whose, essentially guild, concerns derive more from a desire to minimize competition and protect income than to protect the public.

Despite attempts by their competitors to limit their activities, emergent health professionals invariably achieve expansion of their scope of practice. These advancements may occur for a variety of reasons, including evidence of a growing science base for the profession or manifest demonstrations of competence by members of that profession to sanctioners of care. Very often, however, such changes are a direct result of pressure for reform originating either with the public (in the cause of freedom of choice of provider) or from the professions themselves (in the form of self-advocacy or lobbying). While the evidence for the appropriateness of expanding the scope of practice in particular instances may be compelling, it is political pressures which are most influential in determining whether or not legislatures decide to initiate change.

Inadequacies of Legislation

A brief review of licensing and related legislation applying to psychologists in California makes clear why such legislation is inadequate for ensuring competence and appropriate professional behaviors. The basic licensing law, enacted in California in 1967 (Business and Professions Code, Section 2900 et seq.), requires an appropriate doctorate and two years of supervised experience, one of them post-doctoral. Other laws impose more stringent standards in certain situations. For example, hospital medical staff membership requires psychologists to have at least two years clinical experience in a licensed health facility (Health and Safety Code, 1316.5), and certain court services, such as certification for involuntary admission, require a psychologist to have at least five years of post-graduate experience in the diagnosis and treatment of emotional and mental disorders (e.g., Penal Code, 1027). Other regulation delimits which professions may engage in what kind of professional activities in particular settings. Thus, within the Department of Corrections, mental health treatment or diagnostic services must be supervised by a psychiatrist or psychologist (Penal Code, 5079).

As can be seen from these examples, statutory or regulatory authorization and limitation are common well beyond the basic licensure law. The purpose of post-basic licensure standards, or the restriction of certain functions to specified professions, is to provide a general public assurance that the professional services can be reliably performed. In fact, as can also be seen from the examples, there is little reason to believe that, even in the aggregate, these laws serve the purpose of ensuring anything whatsoever about the actual professional performance of providers. What such regulation achieves, however, is the (not always unintended) consequence of reducing competition by limiting access to the marketplace.

Overholser and Fine (1990) conclude that incompetence among mental health professionals is due to lack of knowledge, inadequate clinical skills, poor judgment, and debilitating personal attributes. The mere possession of a license provides no assurance to sanctioners or consumers that the practitioner will remain current with professional developments, will continue to be clinically skilled, or will maintain personal stability. With the exception of post-graduate specialty accreditation or certification, however, little if any ongoing monitoring bears on the professional behaviors of licensed providers. Post-graduate specialty boards are broadly recognized in medicine but less firmly endorsed by psychology and social work. In psychology, for example, the decision to seek such credentailing is voluntary. Boards of this kind provide a post-graduate, post-licensure, in-depth evaluation process developed and conducted by peers. They are the only formal post-licensure examinations now offered, and these procedures constitute the sole instance of formal evaluation of clinical competencies in the life of the relatively small proportion of clinical professionals who submit to this process.

Many states do maintain continuing education requirements which are presumed to ensure ongoing "upgrading" of relevant skills and knowledge of licensed professionals. Unfortunately, such mechanisms generally focus on the process (attendance), not the outcome (what was learned) of educational experiences.

Any potential that licensure laws have for holding the licensee accountable for professional services rendered is generally unrealized, since the mechanisms for monitoring and acting upon public complaints have been shown to be ineffective. The enforcement activities of licensing boards too often appear to emphasize the protection of the profession rather than that of the public. Breakdowns in physician discipline in California by the Medical Board are illustrative of self-serving guild interests which are counter to the spirit of public accountability (Fellmuth, 1989). It is noteworthy that, prior to managed care, and to the extent that this accountability role was fulfilled by any entity, it was more often manifest in the civil court process in the ultimate context of malpractice litigation.

Peer Review and the Law

Peer review has long been accepted by most professions, particularly those involved in health care, as the only legitimate mechanism for making judgments about competence of clinicians or quality of services. At the same time, this mechanism is perceived by many clinicians as an unwarranted intrusion into the provider-patient relationship, a challenge to their competence, a threat to confidentiality, an external compromising factor in the finely-wrought therapeutic process, and, lastly, one which may set external and essentially *ad hoc* limits or conditions on what is felt by many within the provider community to be the provider's legitimate and exclusive role in the determination of parameters of care.

Partly because negative findings by peer reviewers may have significant negative—and unwelcome—consequences for the provider, peer review has traditionally been an under-utilized accountability mechanism. It is also true that providers themselves tend to be uncomfortable in the role of clinical adjudication. The loss of facility "privileges" or vulnerability to malpractice litigation as a result of peer review judgments are very likely to bring threats of legal action from the person whose work has been reviewed adversely. Because of this, the only way peer review could ever become a useful tool was for governments to legislate protection for those engaging in this activity. Such legislation, in general, ensures reviewer anonymity, protects the process from legal discovery, and provides immunity from civil liability to formally constituted peer review groups. Legislation also often applies conditions on such protection— for example, that reviewers act in good faith and without malice.

The removal from discovery aspect limits potential future litigation. Thus it is that the direct interests of the patient, the practitioner, the peer reviewer, the payer, and the attorney are placed, as it were, in abeyance by state law so that the public interest may not only be served but also be seen to be served.

An excellent summary of California's law on peer review is found in Matchett v. Superior Court (1974) 40 Cal. App.3d 623, in which a medical malpractice plaintiff sought the records of various hospital peer review committees:

> ... medical staff committees bear delegated responsibility for the competence of staff practitioners, [and] the quality of in-hospital medical care depends heavily upon the committee members' frankness in evaluating their associates' medical skills and their objectivity in regulating staff privileges. Although

composed of volunteer professionals, these committees are affected with a strong element of public interest.

California law recognizes this public interest by endowing the practitioner-members of hospital staff committees with a measure of immunity from damage claims arising from committee activities [citations omitted]. Evidence Code Section 1157 expresses a legislative judgment that the public interest in medical staff candor extends beyond damage immunity and requires a degree of confidentiality . . . Section 1157 was enacted upon the theory that external access to peer investigations conducted by staff committees stifles candor and inhibits objectivity. It evinces a legislative judgment that the quality of in-hospital medical practice will be elevated by armoring staff inquiries with a measure of confidentiality.

This confidentiality exacts a social cost because it impairs malpractice plaintiffs' access to evidence. In a damage suit for in-hospital malpractice against doctor or hospital or both, unavailability of recorded evidence of incompetence might seriously jeopardize or even prevent the plaintiff's recovery. Section 1157 represents a legislative choice between competing public concerns. It embraces the goal of medical staff candor at the cost of impairing plaintiffs' access to evidence.

The purpose of public protection is augmented by a related peer review statute which requires that adverse peer review findings be reported to relevant licensing boards so that appropriate disciplinary action may be undertaken (Business and Professions Code 800). Similarly, Section 805 of the Business and Professions Code requires peer review bodies to submit reports to the appropriate licensing agency whenever staff privileges, membership, or employment is terminated or curtailed for a "medical disciplinary cause or reason."

In response to the growing phenomenon in which hospitals permitted practitioners to resign rather than discipline them for fear of retaliatory lawsuits, Civil Code Section 43.97 was enacted in 1986, to hold that the reviewers and facility shall be liable only for economic damages, but otherwise enjoy immunity. These provisions apply to professional societies (eg., ethics committee of a state professional association), professional licensing boards, professional peer review committees, and review committees of local mental health programs in addition to hospital medical staff.

In 1982, to encourage price competition in health care, the California legislature amended the Insurance Code, Section 10133 to allow insurers to contract directly with providers at discounted rates. All such contracts were required to include programs for the

. . . continuous review of the quality of care, performance of . . . personnel, utilization of services and facilities and costs, by professionally recognized

> unrelated third parties utilizing in the case of professional providers similarly licensed providers. . . . All provisions of the laws . . . relating to immunity from liability and discovery privileges for . . . peer review shall apply to the licensed providers performing (these) activities.

This was to be the entree for peer review in what would essentially become managed care.

Problems in Implementing Peer Review

A particular deficiency of the current statutory scheme in California is the absence of a legal requirement for private peer review bodies (e.g., professional societies) to report to the responsible regulatory agency. As a result, there have been few such reports and rarely any timely disciplinary action by the relevant board consequent upon the receipt of such reports (Fellmuth, 1989). There are other reasons for the underutilization of peer review, the most critical of which is the lack of a structure to support the process for professionals in traditional independent practice. And, of course, for peer review to work, a prevailing pattern of practice has to be manifest.

Clearly, some kind of professional review mechanism is a critical element in managed care. While previous efforts by legislatures to encourage the effective use of this strategy have not succeeded, the pragmatic need for professional judgment in many aspects of services is making expert review a mandatory instrument in the armamentarium of managed care companies. To the extent that such review is able constructively to intercede to improve the quality of services before regulatory intervention becomes necessary, it fulfills a preventive purpose. The challenge for managed care, therefore, is to establish structures and mechanisms to enable the process to work appropriately.

Judgments about Quality

Judgments about health services can be viewed from the perspective of quantity or intensity of services utilized, cost of those services, or characteristics of the treatment episode, both process and outcome. Too commonly in managed care, a utilization review or cost focus has been substituted for an outcome, or quality focus. This is largely due to the lack of appropriate professional involvement in the actual decision-making process and in the structuring of the review process itself.

This inappropriate review focus is revealed in mechanisms such as a requirement for review of outpatient services at established points (e.g., every tenth session) without regard to the severity or complexity of the presenting condition, characteristics of the treatment plan, or other information about typical patterns of utilization. Such techniques may be convenient for payers, but they are likely to be clinically irrelevant and aggravating in the extreme to practitioners. They may even be cost-ineffective, if the cost of review exceeds the cost of services forgone. Finally, they are not in any consistent way associated with improvements in the clinical status or welfare of clients.

Case-specific judgments about quality of care should be made by a professional. So, too, should judgments about the structure of review and monitoring programs used in managed care programs. Only clinicians are able to balance the clinical and financial realities of a service delivery system. The individual reviewer must bring clinical judgment to bear as well as consider evidence from empirical research about preferred patterns of services and typical patterns of service observed in relevant benefit plans.

For example, data from the Civilian Health and Medical Program of the Uniformed Services (CHAMPUS) indicates that, while the average number of outpatient mental health visits per year for CHAMPUS beneficiaries was 9.7, nearly a fifth (19.2%) of the users had but a single visit, and 30.7% had two visits. Only 1% of users had as many as 20 visits and only .1% had 52 visits. The CHAMPUS Reform Initiative calls for review after the sixth and every subsequent ten visits. Under this plan, at the first two review points, 55.6% and 80.3% of users, respectively, would have completed treatment. Under the standard CHAMPUS plan, review occurs after the twenty-third outpatient visit, at which point 88.1% have completed their treatment.

It is obvious that a review of all treatment plans makes no sense, given that almost half of all utilizers of service will cease treatment after two sessions. At the same time, if a goal of the review system is a quality assurance one, delaying the first review to the 24th session means that only about 10% of cases will ever receive any scrutiny. Too little review not only defeats the quality assurance purpose of a monitoring program, it also encourages fraud and abuse by providers.

Conclusion

Efforts to manage care are only feasible because of the growing scientific base of behavioral health services. Because of this, managed systems must depend upon expert professional opinion to apply what is known about the appropriate utilization of behavioral health interventions in individual episodes of care and to create the systems through which care will be managed. The latter function would include, for example, the development of practice guidelines which supplement judgment in the review process, rules for implementation of these guidelines, and procedures for giving feedback to providers. In short, professional judgment must be the primary factor in balancing the cost needs of the review program against the clinical needs of patients and clients. Professional judgment is, however, only one necessary factor in the development of appropriate structures and processes for managing care.

In some ways, the accountability wheel has come full circle. For decades clinical practice was characterized by a strictly non-interventionist approach by sanctioners such as governments and payers. In the absence of a developed consumerist movement, practice was left to the professions; the professional associations needed only pay lip service to their commitment to practice standards development and implementation to mollify any residual governmental concerns about public accountability. As egregious instances of poor quality clinical practice surfaced, governments increasingly resorted to regulatory legislation to "protect the public." And some of these regulations referred to the formal peer review process by way of inducing the professions to police themselves. With consumerism gaining strength, the public's interest increasingly came to be represented in litigation. However personally satisfying the few judgments which found in the plaintiff's favor, the tort focus of the civil courts could not in any way have been a substitute for quality assurance in the public interest. It is laborious, non-systematic, and hideously expensive; its effect on practice patterns encourages "defensive" care, not appropriate care.

It has been a revolution of the payers—of the large employers—which has driven the managed care movement and, as we have seen, the case management companies initially sought to "manage" exclusively through services manipulation. Only fairly recently has the industry begun to do what neither the nation's legislatures nor the professional associations have succeeded in doing: develop *systems* of care in which the consensual judgment of practicing clinicians is the critical factor in the quality equation. As we have also seen, the focus of peer review itself has changed. From a formalistic approach far removed in time from the clinical decision process, it is emerging as a critical tool for systems quality improvement. In its new form, at its best, it is site-based, emphasizes consensual judgments arrived at by a collegial process of inter-professional communication, and is often multi-disciplinary, not peer-focused. In essence, it has become consultative and responsive—a far more effective mechanism for protecting the interests of the consumer than external regulatory safeguards possessing limited essential force.

Thus it has been that a rapidly developing, essentially pragmatic industry has come to co-opt peer review as a mechanism for clinical quality assurance. Once used mainly in the context of government-initiated external regulation, local and consultative processes of inter-professional consensus are increasingly used by managed care companies as a central mechanism for clinical quality assessment and improvement. Of particular interest is the fact that the managed behavioral health care industry itself, rather than the professional associations or academia, is most associated with this development.

REFERENCES

Devine, E. and Cook, T. (1983). A meta-analysis of effects of psycho-educational interventions on length of post-surgical hospital stay. *Nursing Research, 32,* 267–274.

Fellmuth, R. (1989). Physician discipline in California: A code blue emergency. *The California Regulatory Law Reporter, 9,* 1–19.

Follette, W. and Cummings, N. (1967). Psychiatric services and medical utilization in a prepaid health plan setting. *Medical Care, 5,* 25–35.

Fordyce, W. (1988). Pain and Suffering: A reappraisal. *American Psychologist, 43,* 276–283.

Gruen, W. (1975). Effects of brief psychotherapy during the hospitalization period on the recovery process in heart attacks. *Journal of Consulting and Clinical Psychology, 43,* 223–232.

Jones, K. and Vischi, T. (1979). The impact of alcohol, drug abuse and mental health treatment on medical care utilization: A review of the research literature. *Medical Care, 17,* No. 12 Supplement.

Mumford, E., Schlesinger, H., and Glass, G. (1984). The effects of psychological intervention on recovery from surgery and heart attacks: An analysis of the literature. *American Journal of Public Health, 72,* 141–151.

Overholser, J. and Fine, M. (1990). Defining the boundaries of professional competence: Managing subtle cases of incompetence. *Professional Psychology: Research and Practice, 24,* 462–469.

Schlesinger, H., Mumford, E., Glass, G., Patrick, C., and Sharfstein, S. (1983). Mental health treatment and medical care utilization in a fee-for-service system: Outpatient mental health treatment following the onset of a chronic disease. *American Journal of Public Health, 73,* 422–429.

Smith, M. and Glass, G. (1977). Meta-analysis of psychotherapy outcome studies, *American Psychologist, 32,* 752–760.

U.S. Office of Technology Assessment (1978). Assessing the Efficacy and Safety of Medical Technologies, No. 052-003-00593-0. Washington D.C.: U.S. Government Printing Office.

Wiens, A. and Dörken, H. (1986). Establishing and enforcing standards to assure professional competency. In Dörken and Associates (Eds.), *Professional Psychology in Transition: Meeting Today's Challenges.* San Francisco: Jossey-Bass, 174–199.

PART IV
ASSESSING AND IMPROVING THE
QUALITY OF SERVICES

PART IV: INTRODUCTORY NOTE

Historically, quality assurance (QA) in health services has been viewed as a necessary inconvenience, with ritualistic compliance generally regarded as adequate. It is only with the development and marketing of managed care that quality has been awarded the position of a high priority, high profile concern.

One reason for the ascendancy of QA is defensiveness on the part of managed delivery organizations themselves. They implement QA activities to reassure consumers, purchasers, and providers that the cost-saving focus of managed systems does not compromise the quality of care. A second reason is that QA is considered a useful marketing device in the competitive world of for-profit health care.

Not only do managed systems provide significant incentive for improving quality (i.e., increased sales), they also provide the necessary access to data about services and the system control needed to implement quality improvement activities. There is no doubt that these programs provide the best available setting for the implementation of effective QA systems. As Shueman and Troy discuss in Chapter 8, quality monitoring as well as quality improvement are difficult if not impossible in context of traditional, uncontrolled, service delivery. As the authors suggest, however, the real challenge to these organizations is to involve all stakeholders in the process of defining, measuring, and improving quality. Until such collaborative efforts occur, quality assurance activities in managed care will, to too great an extent, resemble the traditional and ineffective external regulatory approaches to QA.

One of the most important aspects of the development of QA in managed care has been the attempt to ensure that services provided are consistent with service delivery patterns that empirical research has suggested are effective. This has been referred to as "bringing research into practice." In Chapter 9, Shueman and Troy discuss one manifestation of this strategy: the application of empirically-based practice guidelines.

The introduction of practice guidelines has been especially critical to the development of managed behavioral health care. Quality of care can never be effectively addressed if there is no agreement within the provider community about what the process of care should be, and behavioral health service providers have been particularly resistant to any attempt to gain consensus on preferred treatments. Unfortunately, however, practice guidelines have not evolved from the provider community, and therein lies one of their significant faults. At the same time, they do offer a starting point for discussion about how services should be delivered. Such an *informed* discussion has traditionally been studiously avoided by the mental health provider community.

Chapter 8

QUALITY ASSURANCE IN MANAGED SYSTEMS

Sharon A. Shueman and Warwick G. Troy

Recent years have witnessed a significant increase in the amount of effort devoted to strategies for containing costs in all areas of health care, including behavioral health. These efforts have brought with them concerns about the effects that cost-containment activities might have on the quality of care. Furthermore, managed care organizations are "selling" quality. It has become a commodity which they are attempting to use for competitive advantage. For these reasons, quality assurance activities are increasing in perceived as well as genuine importance. For perhaps the first time in history, significant resources are being allocated to develop and maintain effective QA mechanisms in all health service systems.

The main focus of this chapter is on the design of quality assurance strategies for managed behavioral health care systems. An adequate QA program must above all explicitly recognize and address the complex nature of a managed service delivery system. This requires a comprehensive QA program which reflects perspectives of multiple stakeholders (at a minimum, patients and their families, providers, payers, and system administrators); which focuses on multiple aspects of clinical services, case management, and administration; and, finally, which uses a range of objective and subjective data elements and multiple data sources in the assessment of quality.

This chapter is not intended to be a primer on QA. It is intended to give the reader an adequate basis for understanding the applications of the principles discussed here. Much of the chapter reflects a relatively traditional QA approach. Traditional QA provides the theoretical and practical bases for all current quality-focused activities, whether they are described as quality assurance or, in more popular jargon, as quality management, quality improvement, or quality enhancement. At the same time, the chapter also includes a discussion of ways in which the applications of QA have been influenced by these more recent approaches to quality, particularly the principles of total quality management (Deming, 1982; Walton, 1989) and continuous quality improvement (Berwick, 1989).

WHAT IS QUALITY ASSURANCE?

The standard definition of quality assurance in medical care comes from Donabedian (1980) who describes it as consisting of two components:

1. *quality assessment:* measuring the extent to which the care satisfies previously established standards for quality; and
2. *feedback:* providing information to the system which is necessary to implement efforts to correct deficiencies identified by the quality assessment process.

In other words, *quality **assurance** results when findings from quality **assessment** activities are used to guide efforts to improve the system.* A set of activities can not be classified as quality assurance unless it includes activities focused on both assessment and feedback aimed at quality improvement.

A QA program is continuous. Indeed, Donabedian's (1980) model may be characterized as circular, with sequential and repetitive processes of assessment, feedback, and reassessment to determine the effects of improvement efforts. Over time, the foci of QA activities in any organization will almost certainly change, as different aspects of the system are targeted to receive more or less scrutiny and effort, but the service system as a whole is never considered "good enough" to warrant discontinuation of the QA process.

Defining Quality

Judgments about quality are made with respect to criteria and standards. Criteria are merely elements which are observed, counted, and measured in the process of assessing quality (Donabedian, 1982). Length of stay, for example, is one criterion used in the evaluation of hospital care. Use of medication is another. Standard connotes a "*desired* achievable (rather than *observed*) performance or value" with regard to a criterion (Slee, 1974, p. 100). In other words, standards describe the level at which the system should perform. A standard would specify a desired length of stay for a given diagnosis or optimal use of a specific drug for a specific condition.

Adequate quality services are those which are determined by the quality assessment process to satisfy the established standards. In other words: *quality is defined as adherence to standards established for the service system.* It follows that the definition of quality varies across service systems according to both the criteria (what is focused on) and the standards (what level of performance is desired) applying within each service environment.

Multiple Perspectives on Quality

The criteria from which standards are derived reflect what is important to or valued by various stakeholder groups. This means that quality is an expression of values of the various groups of persons involved with the administration, financing, delivery, and consumption of the services. In addition to patients and their families or significant others, these groups include, providers, payers (who are often employers), and case managers.

The inclusion of multiple perspectives helps ensure the "constructive tension" that is the natural safeguard in any system. For example, any observer of health care knows that one of the most common struggles in service delivery is between the providers, whose primary concern is that patients receive "enough" service, and the payers, for whom the primary concerns are the cost and, perhaps secondarily, the cost-effectiveness of the services provided by the system. A tension between these two groups is one of the factors which helps ensure that patients are neither under- nor over-served.

Consider some examples from four perspectives which exist in any managed system. Providers in such a system may value factors such as ease of access to competent, clinically experienced case managers which makes it easier for them to work within the constraints imposed by the managed system. From the perspective of this stakeholder group, then, criteria should address issues such as minimum qualifications and competencies of case managers, their availability to providers phoning for pre-certification, and the manner in which they relate to providers.

Employers purchasing a managed program may be concerned about the cost-effectiveness of the services which they purchase as well as the level of satisfaction of the employees and their dependents who use the services. Criteria of importance to employers, therefore, might address appropriateness of practice patterns (i.e., adherence to "practice guidelines" [Eddy, 1990b]) and cost issues such as intensity and frequency of services in a given treatment episode. They would also address outcome as assessed both objectively, using standardized measures, and subjectively, by patients.

Patients may be primarily concerned about access to care and the capacity of providers in the system to help them solve their problems. Criteria relevant to the former concern might address geographical distribution of providers in the network, or length of time between intake and first service. Criteria relevant to the latter concern could include patient satisfaction as reflected on surveys, or change in patients' level of functioning as reflected on standardized assessment instruments.

In addition to cost-effectiveness of providers, system administrators may value providers' willingness to cooperate with case managers and to satisfy the administrative requirements of the managed system. Relevant criteria might reflect case managers' assessments of their interactions with network providers, or the providers' level of cooperation in submitting appropriate clinical information.

Multiple Measures and Data Sources

Just as multiple perspectives must be included in assessment of quality, so too must multiple data sources define the bases for making decisions about quality. For example, asking a patient about the effect of services he or she received is a legitimate measure of service quality. A better measure of quality of outcome is achieved, however, by also seeking information on effect from the patient's parent, spouse, or significant other. Similarly, while it is reasonable to ask clinicians to rate the impact of their services on individual patients, it is also important to use a more objective measure, such as standardized problem checklist or level of functioning scale, for a second clinical perspective.

Consider, for example, the question of the quality of the outcome of an episode of behavioral health services. Some possible foci for criteria are:

- The patient's evaluation of the outcome of treatment;
- Evaluation of outcome by a member of the patient's family;
- The service provider's evaluation of outcome;
- Change in the patient's score on a standardized assessment instrument (e.g., Beck Depression Inventory);
- The patient's level of functioning three months after discharge;
- Whether or not the patient makes an unplanned request for subsequent treatment.

While each indicator may, in and of itself, validly reflect some aspect of the quality of the services, a single indicator generally does not tell the whole quality story. This becomes clearer in context of a specific example.

> Simon entered treatment (individual psychotherapy with a psychologist) for major depression. His condition improved after four months, as evidenced by change score on the Beck Depression Inventory. His discharge from treatment after 5 months was a joint decision by Simon and his therapist, since both were satisfied with the outcome of the treatment. However, despite the fact that Simon had reported to his provider that his depression had been recurrent over the prior four years, the therapist did not seriously consider sending him to a psychiatrist for consultation regarding the possible use of maintenance medication. (Empirical research indicates that the use of such medication may be advisable for patients with more than two prior episodes of major depression [Kupfer & Frank, 1987]). Seven months later, Simon returned to treatment experiencing another major depressive episode.

In Simon's case, indicators 1, 3, and 4, above, would have reflected good quality of care at discharge. At the same time, indicators 5 (perhaps) and 6 (certainly) would have brought into question the quality of the services.

His return to treatment does not necessarily mean that Simon received poor quality care. He may not have been helped by medication. If he would have benefited from it, however, the extra cost of a psychiatric consultation would have been a cost-effective investment. From the perspectives of the payer and the system administrators as well as Simon, then, it would have been preferable for the therapist at least to consider the use of medication. The quality issue here is that the provider, apparently, was not aware of the scientific evidence relevant to drug treatment of the type of depression with which Simon presented.

Levels of Quality

The use of standards implies a desired or expected level of performance. Each service system sets its own level, and it follows that quality is not an absolute concept. There are two general approaches to setting the expected level of performance: to establish what is minimally acceptable ("basement" standards), or to focus on the level of service the service system aspires to achieve ("aspirational" or optimal standards).

Adoption of minimum standards suggests that the primary concerns of the service system are reduction of risk and avoidance of liability. Since an incremental increase in the number or level of standards is accompanied by an increase in the cost of implementing them, organizations opting for a minimalist approach set standards no higher than is deemed necessary to reduce risk and potential liability to an acceptable level.

Adoption of optimal standards, on the other hand, is a reflection of the organization's intent to continually improve the quality of its services. This is quite consistent with more recent approaches to quality in which the explicit assumption is that all standards should be set at a 100% level. In other words, the ultimate goal of a system taking such an approach is to achieve perfection. What this means in practice is that the system never stops trying to improve.

Criteria which Define Quality

Criteria defining quality may focus on any of three aspects of a service system: *structure, process,* or *outcome* (Donabedian, 1980). Structure refers to the attributes of a service setting, including those of material and human resources. Process refers to what goes on within and between patients and service providers. Finally, outcome refers to the effects of service on patients. Historically, criteria in health care have focused predominantly on structure and process. Until recently, for example, state and federal licensing bodies and accreditation organizations such as the Joint Commission for the Accreditation of Healthcare Organizations (JCAHO) have focused almost exclusively on these two dimensions of the service system.

In managed systems, structural criteria focus on factors such as: training, experience, competencies, and malpractice history of providers; training and experience of case managers; and the licensing and accreditation status of hospitals or other organized care settings. These criteria are not substantially different from structural criteria traditionally used in non-managed systems, although some seemingly minor differences are significant. For example, in some managed programs criteria specify that it is desirable for network providers have one or more of the following types of work experiences:

- Community mental health center, other community-based agency, or Veterans Administration facility;
- QA or utilization review committee service in an organized care setting;
- Health services administration; and
- Program evaluation or applied clinical research.

The rationale for this is that such experiences give behavioral health providers a broader perspective on clinical services and an appreciation of the need for accountability.

Process criteria in managed care also tend to be broader in scope than those used traditionally (for example, in institutional accreditation programs). While addressing traditional factors such as clinical documentation, committee activities, program evaluation, and adherence to policies and procedures, criteria in managed systems heavily emphasize the types of criteria generally referred to as "practice guidelines" (Shueman & Troy, 1993). The promulgation of this type of empirically-based criteria has been one of the most significant contributions of the managed approach to health services.

Outcome criteria address issues such as patient satisfaction, change as reflected on standardized assessment instruments, change as judged by patients or family members, and recidivism or relapse (e.g., a second episode of hospitalization or return to substance use following a drug rehabilitation program). Outcome criteria have been neglected in health care because of the perceived difficulties in defining and measuring outcome, but also because service providers' have been unwilling to be held accountable for outcome. The typical arguments against accountability have been: (1) too many patient factors (e.g., motivation for treatment, compliance) and environmental events (e.g., unfortunate family situation, tragic life events) which are outside of the control of the therapist could negatively affect outcome; and (2) it is difficult to state in measurable or observable terms what the goals of treatment are and, hence, it is not possible for someone outside the therapeutic relationship to know when they are achieved.

The new emphasis on accountability in health care brought about by payers has given treatment outcomes assessment a featured place in quality assurance. This has been particularly challenging to service providers, many of whom for the first time are being asked to work within a time-limited, problem-focused treatment model. In many cases this has necessitated a change in attitude as well as acquisition of new skills.

Two Types of Criteria

Criteria may be either *explicit* or *implicit.* Explicit criteria are usually documented as formal criteria sets and used in institutional (hospital) settings. The criteria discussed so far in this chapter are explicit. Implicit criteria are manifest only in the judgments of professionals such as peer reviewers or members of a QA Committee.

Explicit criteria are more easily applied than those which are implicit, since the former are more likely to be observable or measurable. Their relative ease of application means that they are typically used to review large numbers of cases with the objective of identifying "outliers"—episodes of care which exhibit significant variation from a criterion and, therefore, are believed to warrant greater scrutiny or corrective action. Once identified, these cases may used to develop profiles of providers, institutions, diagnostic groups, etc. to determine foci for additional quality assessment or quality improvement activities. These profiles may take the many forms, such as numerical reports or graphical representations of data.

Profiles generally do not provide definitive answers about quality of care. For example, profiles of a group of drug rehabilitation programs may suggest particularly good outcomes—as reflected in very low relapse—for one drug rehabilitation program and very poor outcome for several others. Such a finding does not necessarily mean that the former program is excellent and the latter several are of poor quality. It may be that the program with the better outcomes tends to serve the types of patients who are less likely to relapse. Similarly, one or more of the latter programs may specialize in the more difficult patients.

To determine more definitively which programs provide better quality services, it would be helpful to look at profiles of these programs regarding other criteria—for example, the percent of patients actually completing treatment. Ultimately, however, valid decisions about quality would necessitate review of individual episodes of care provided within these programs, examining both the types of patients being treated and the characteristics of the treatment episodes. This process would be based upon the application of implicit criteria—the professional clinical judgments of the individuals conducting the reviews. These types of judgments are the final arbiters of quality of care in specific applications of service (Eddy, 1990a).

The Quality Assurance Activity

Quality assurance has, historically, been accorded low status in health care, perhaps even more so in behavioral health than in medical-surgical care. While organized care settings such as hospitals and community mental health centers invariably maintain QA programs, such programs have usually been engaged in for two reasons, neither of which reflects a valuing of QA.

The first reason is that external sanctioning agencies such as JCAHO, state licensing authorities, and third-party payers such as Medicare have demanded that service organizations develop and maintain QA programs. If an organization does not maintain a QA program, it will not be licensed or accredited and, therefore, will lose access to significant funding such as Medicare reimbursement.

A second reason QA has been undertaken is to protect against legal liability. Service organizations orient QA activities toward minimizing the risk that harm could come to a patient as a result of the system's inadequacies. An example of such an activity is the almost universal practice of reviewing "adverse events" (e.g., drug overdose, suicide attempt, discharge against medical advice) to determine whether a system inadequacy contributed to the event and, if so, what could be done to minimize the probability of a recurrence.

In summary, organizations have traditionally done QA because they were forced to. If the external pressures and threats were not there, QA would not have been accorded even the grudging attention which was frequently the case.

Until the introduction of managed care, it was not unusual for lower status professionals, generally nurses, to constitute QA committees in organized care settings, and the work of these committees was generally unknown outside of the committee membership. Their formal objectives tended to emphasize detection and correction of deficiencies which had already occurred in individual clinical episodes, but their efforts to correct the deficiencies were most often ignored by those professionals— often doctors—whose work was the subject of the quality assessment activities. This focus on quality assessment by lower status providers almost guaranteed that little system action resulted as a function of the feedback. In other words, little quality assurance resulted from quality assessment activities.

Independent Providers and QA

QA has been even less relevant to independent practitioners than it has been to institutions. Prior to managed care, behavioral health professionals functioning outside of organized care settings rarely engaged in QA activities. Few were introduced to principles or practices of QA in their graduate training programs. Therefore, even if they wished to engage in QA, they had little capacity to do so without the support of the formal structures provided by organized care settings. At most, these professionals participated in case conferences or clinical supervision, activities which often satisfied their need to feel as though they were engaging in quality assurance activities, but which generally proved to be more intellectual exercise or posturing than quality assurance. It was only with the appearance of the forerunners of managed care programs, such as the CHAMPUS Peer Review Program begun in 1979 (Penner, 1993), that substantial numbers of independent mental health practitioners became aware of the concept of quality assurance and made their first halting attempts to comply with accountability requirements.

Integration of QA into Managed Care

The greatest strength of the managed care approach is its requirement that health services be delivered in context of a **system.** It is only in this context that the quality of health services can be effectively monitored and effective strategies for improvement be implemented. With the notable exception of group or staff model (i.e., closed panel) health maintenance organizations, health care has traditionally not been delivered systematically in any environment.

In the typical example prior to managed care, health services were provided by an independent practitioner, program, or institution and paid for on a fee-for-service basis by a third-party payer with which the provider had no formal connection other than as a vendor. In such a situation, it was not clear who was responsible for detecting and correcting compromises to quality. For example, the traditional "system" had no effective mechanism for ascertaining or dealing with circumstances such as: the patient being lost to follow up in the transition from inpatient to outpatient services; the patient "doctor shopping" in attempts to find a provider who is willing to prescribe the type of medication which the patient wants but may not benefit from; the patient being uninformed about a low cost, appropriate community-based support service; or the patient receiving services from an incompetent provider.

The systems created by managed care organizations in theory provide excellent opportunities to detect and correct or prevent these problems of continuity of care. They provide structures for designating a single individual—the case manager—to be responsible for care, and a data monitoring system to track patients through the service system. Perhaps most importantly, since the case manager is basically the agent of the payer, he or she also has the authority to ensure that corrective actions are taken.

Desired Characteristics of QA System

The critical characteristics of an ideal QA system are the same, whether it is implemented within or outside of a managed care context. The following are proposed as the four most important factors in the development of such a system.

Comprehensiveness

Managed care systems are complex, and any attempt at QA must subsume all aspects of the system which could potentially influence the services received by the beneficiaries. Managed systems are composed of three major elements which constitute foci for QA activities: the *clinical services,* the *case management services,* and the *program administration.*

In addition to subsuming these three critical aspects of the service system, an adequate QA program must also focus on the three service dimensions: structure, process, and outcome. Figure 1 provides examples of structure, process, and outcome foci and related data sources for QA activities in a managed care program.

Figure 1 includes examples which look very familiar to the eye of a health services professional experienced in QA. For example, subsumed under structural criteria are review of credentials for professionals and licensing or accreditation status for institutions. Process criteria address clinical audits, administrative audits, and patient evaluation of services. Outcome criteria address assessment of patient improvement, patient satisfaction surveys, and review of adverse events.

Other elements listed on Figure 1 represent aspects of QA which, if not unique to managed care, have not typically been foci in QA. One example is expert panel reviews of the clinical criteria which form the basis of the system's practice guidelines. Traditionally, institutions and programs adopted externally developed standardized criteria sets. Managed care companies now maintain their own empirically based sets derived from reviews of the empirical literature and consultation with experts. It is likely that some of these companies will even be establishing research programs, either independently or in collaboration with uni-

Figure 1

Selected Foci and Data Sources for Quality Assurance Activities

System Component	Focus	Data Source
DIMENSION OF CARE: **STRUCTURE**		
Case Management	Qualifications of case managers	Credentials
Clinical Service Provision	Institution and organization capabilities	Program description, license, accreditation status
	Appropriateness of clinical criteria	Expert panel reviews
DIMENSION OF CARE: **PROCESS**		
Eligibility/claims	Timeliness, accuracy of eligibility verification	Monthly activity report
	Completion of transfer to case management	Monthly activity report
Case Management	Appropriateness of referral	Case manager profile Provider evaluation of case manager
	Interaction with patient	Patient satisfaction survey
	Accuracy and completeness of documentation	Administrative audit
	Appropriateness of application of criteria	Clinical case audit
Clinical Services Provision	Appropriateness of treatment plan	Case manager evaluation of episode of care Clinical case audit
	Adherence to administrative requirements	Administrative case audit
	Interaction with case manager	Case manager evaluation of episode of care
DIMENSION OF CARE: **OUTCOME**		
Case Management	Adverse occurrences	Case manager profile Occurrence record
	Outcome of appeals	Case manager profile
	Patient satisfaction	Patient survey
Clinical Services Provision	Patient improvement	Level of functioning change score
	Readmissions	Provider profile
	Patient satisfaction	Patient satisfaction survey

versities, to further develop and refine criteria. With practice guide-lines playing such a major role in the management of the service system, it is critical that their validity and appropriateness be constantly re-evaluated.

A second example of these "new" elements is the determination of the timeliness and accuracy of eligibility verification. Since financing and service delivery are integrated in managed systems, access to services is a direct function of eligibility determination. A false positive determination may result in an unexpected, perhaps substantial, financial cost to a patient or loss to the provider; a false negative may cause a critical delay or even prevent access to services.

An additional component of critical importance to the quality of the service system is the *benefit.* The benefit is a written statement which specifies the covered conditions, types of care, eligible providers, and conditions of payment which apply to a defined beneficiary group. One of the most common criticisms of managed as well as non-managed systems of financing behavioral health services is that the range of appropriate alternatives are not included in the benefit, or that the financing scheme encourages use of inappropriate and cost-ineffective alternatives. For example, many plans inadvertently encourage the use of inpatient care by providing more generous financing of these services or by failing to include in the benefit cost-effective alternatives such as partial hospitalization and day treatment. An appropriate benefit is necessary to ensure access to appropriate services and, therefore, the structure of the benefit is a legitimate focus for quality assessment.

Support for QA at the Highest Levels

The literature on QA applications provides persuasive evidence that the QA system must have the support of everyone in the organization, including those at the highest levels—the board of directors and chief executives. Furthermore, this support must be reflected in a level of financial resources adequate to ensure quality. The best way to ensure support for QA is to make the quality assurance goals and objectives part of the organization's strategic plan. Statements of what the organization hopes to accomplish vis-à-vis QA need to be phrased in structure, process, and outcome terms with appropriate time lines. The board of directors needs to endorse these statements to ensure that adequate resources will be available to the QA program and that it will be taken seriously by everyone within the organization.

Organizations appear (indeed, must appear) to value QA. The inescapable conclusion, however, is that personnel, systems, and financial resources for quality assurance activities are still inadequately developed in most organizations. Every additional QA activity is a drain on the organization's resources. Since managed care corporations are concerned about the "bottom line," they will not willingly engage in QA activities until they are convinced of their cost-benefit.

Involving Stakeholders in QA Development

All stakeholders have a legitimate role not only in evaluating the quality of services, but also in fashioning the QA system itself. Only with the involvement of all parties can a QA program be developed which will ensure the "constructive tension" necessary to balance the interests of the various stakeholder groups.

Of the four groups, consumers and network providers appear to have been the least involved in the development process. With regard to consumers, there is no obvious barrier to their involvement. There are a multitude of obvious mechanisms, primarily developed in public sector service agencies, to involve consumers, particularly advocacy groups. What seems to be necessary is for managed care organizations to realize the potential importance of consumers' contributions and for payers to insist upon effective involvement of their beneficiaries or appropriate advocate organizations.

The most serious challenge appears to involve providers. Mostly due to historical divisions and antipathy between payers and providers, the latter have been held at "arms length" from the corporate entity which is the managed care system. More often than not system administrators have been satisfied with gaining passive compliance from providers, and the providers themselves have not insisted upon having an active, constructive role in the development of systems. To date most of their energies, and those of their guild-oriented professional associations, appear to have been devoted to trying to defeat the management process.

The involvement of network providers is particularly critical to the development of the technical (clinical) criteria which have such a significant impact on the way services are delivered. The path to achievement of valid and reasonable clinical criteria will be significantly longer and more arduous without the ongoing involvement of providers who are asked to implement the criteria while responding to the exigencies of day-to-day practice.

The Role of a Management Information System

It should be clear from the previous discussions that a QA program can not be effective unless it is structured around a comprehensive computer-based management information system (Rogerson, 1993). The complexity of a managed system, the requirement for close monitoring of large numbers of cases and large amounts of clinical and administrative data, and the need for different stakeholder groups to have access to different types and amounts of data in a timely way all require that an efficient system be maintained.

Recent Advances in the Theory of Quality Assurance

Quality assurance is subject to the influences of major socioeconomic change. The current innovations which are seen to be having significant influence on at least the theory if not the practice of QA activities are *continuous quality improvement* (Berwick, 1989) and *total quality management* (Walton, 1989).

What is New in Quality?

Despite appearances of a revolution in quality assurance, little is really new with "new" approaches to QA in health services. These approaches, exemplified by total quality management, had their origins with industrial quality assurance, and the work of adherents such as Deming (1982) has resulted in significant changes in the industrial environment. Health services personnel observing the radical changes heard the criticisms of the old ways of industrial QA, concluded that these same criticisms applied to QA as typically applied in health services (e.g., externally imposed, adversarial process, driven by inspection), and quickly developed an enthusiasm for applying the new techniques to their own field. What many were unaware of was that the approaches endorsed by the new gurus were not at all inconsistent with approaches put forth by Donabedian (1985) as well as other writers on QA in health services, but not generally implemented appropriately in service delivery settings.

This fact, however, does not diminish the contributions of people like Deming (1982) and his followers, who helped lessen the academic/research mystique which has surrounded QA, particularly in health services. Donabedian's work, for example, is not easy to read and it has generally been distributed in very technical academic publications. Quality assurance has become much more accessible to the "average" reader (see, for example, Berwick, 1991). QA's successes are being well publicized, and, partly for this reason, it has come to be regarded as an activity which *can make a difference.*

Suppose that the new models of quality are better than the old. The question remains: What are the particular strengths of these methods? There have been two major contributions to QA in health services made by the proponents of theories such as total quality management and continuous quality improvement. The first has been the principle that *quality is everyone's business.* In the health services setting this means that QA is no longer to be regarded as an administrative activity or the responsibility of "the nurses on the QA Committee," and no longer is it characterized as adversarial. All participants have been told that they are a critical component in the service system and that the quality of what they do *depends upon and has an impact on* the quality of what everyone else does. In essence, they are all each others' customers. It is an essentially egalitarian philosophy which promotes teamwork and which, if implemented correctly, can successfully engage everyone in the pursuit of quality.

The second contribution of these new theories is the principle that, since we never really know how good we can be, there is little point in setting arbitrary standards which may only act to limit our accomplishments. This approach, embodied in continuous quality improvement, implies that the appropriate standard is perfection. It makes implementation of QA activities more difficult—it is, after all, easier merely to determine whether or not a standard is met. At the same time, it increases the probability that a service system will achieve excellence.

Conclusion

Three statements are axiomatic with regard to any quality assurance program:

- The definition and assessment of quality should reflect the perspectives of multiple stakeholders.
- QA activities should focus on multiple aspects of the service system including structure, process, and outcome, and they should utilize multiple data sources.

• The primary objective of the QA program should be continual improvement in the quality of services.

The new models of managed behavioral health care provide excellent vehicles for developing QA systems which satisfy these three principles. At the same time, it must be said that not all that much has changed in the day-to-day world of quality assessment and quality improvement. Despite claims to the contrary and despite the increasing emphasis on quality, managed care has been driven primarily by cost containment, and managed care companies have been driven by profit. Unless and until these companies are convinced that quality assessment and improvement efforts are positively related to more cost-effective services, the typical QA program will be characterized by the ritualistic compliance which has typified such programs in the past. If this happens, the real potential for managed systems to contribute to the improvement in the quality of health services will go unrealized.

REFERENCES

Berwick, D.M. (1989). Continuous improvement as an ideal in health care. *New England Journal of Medicine, 320,* 53–56.

Berwick, D.M., Godfrey, A.B., & Roessner, J. (1991). *Curing Health Care.* San Francisco: Jossey-Bass.

Deming, W.E. (1982). *Quality, Productivity, and Competitive Position.* Cambridge, MA: Massachusetts Institute of Technology, Center for Advanced Engineering Study.

Donabedian, A. (1980). *Explorations in Quality Assessment and Monitoring. Volume I. The Definition of Quality and Approaches to its Assessment.* Ann Arbor, MI: Health Administration Press.

Donabedian, A. (1982). *Explorations in Quality Assessment and Monitoring. Volume II. Criteria and Standards of Quality.* Ann Arbor, MI: Health Administration Press.

Donabedian, A. (1985). *Explorations in Quality Assessment and Monitoring. Volume III. Methods and Findings of Quality Assessment and Monitoring: An Illustrated Analysis.* Ann Arbor, MI: Health Administration Press.

Eddy, D. (1990a). Anatomy of a decision. *Journal of the American Medical Association, 263,* 441–443.

Eddy, D. (1990b). Practice policies: What are they? *Journal of the American Medical Association, 263,* 877–880.

Kupfer, D.J., & Frank, E. (1987). Relapse in recurrent unipolar depression. *American Journal of Psychiatry, 144,* 86–88.

Penner, N.R. (1994). The road from peer review to managed care: Historical perspective. In S.A. Shueman, W.G. Troy, & S.L. Mayhugh (Eds.), *Managed Behavioral Health Care: An Industry Perspective.* Springfield, Illinois: Charles C Thomas, 29–44.

Rogerson, C.L. (1994). Information system requirements for managed care programs. In S.A. Shueman, W.G. Troy, & S.L. Mayhugh (Eds.), *Managed Behavioral Health Care: An Industry Perspective.* Springfield, Illinois: Charles C Thomas, 193–204.

Shueman, S.A. & Troy, W.G. (1994). The use of practice guidelines in managed behavioral health programs. In S.A. Shueman, W.G. Troy, & S.L. Mayhugh (Eds.), *Managed Behavioral Health Care: An Industry Perspective.* Springfield, Illinois: Charles C Thomas, 149–164.

Slee, V. (1974). PSRO and the hospital's quality control. *Annals of Internal Medicine, 81,* 97–106.

Walton, M. (1989). *The Deming Management Method.* London: W.H. Allen & Co.

Chapter 9

THE USE OF PRACTICE GUIDELINES IN MANAGED BEHAVIORAL HEALTH PROGRAMS

SHARON A. SHUEMAN AND WARWICK G. TROY

Practice guidelines are "recommendations issued for the purpose of influencing decisions about health innovations" (Eddy, 1990d). As conceptualized in this chapter they are statements developed through a formal, organized process which reflect state-of-the-art scientific evidence and expert opinion about efficacy of alternative health care strategies. They are used in context of managed care to assist in making determinations of necessity and appropriateness of services provided through these managed arrangements.

This chapter discusses the nature, uses, and implications of practice guidelines in managed behavioral health programs. We consider the evolution of guidelines and the rationale for their use, we describe current guidelines and their uses in managed care programs, and we speculate about what the future holds for practice guidelines and their ilk.

An Historical Perspective

Criteria, standards, and guidelines intended to influence the technical (Donabedian, 1980) aspects of mental health practice are not new, but within the last decade their basic nature has changed. Health services have always been guided by formal and informal normative statements about the process of clinical care. Generally, they have been manifest in three forms: (1) as information in textbooks; (2) as the acquired wisdom of mental health professionals who would pass this lore on to students and colleagues in context of teaching, supervision, or consultation; and (3) as written criteria sets intended primarily to provide guidance to payers and other sanctioners about what is appropriate. It is this third type of statement which was the precursor of current practice guidelines,

149

and it is with such efforts that we are primarily concerned in the remainder of this chapter.

Guidelines as Norms

What the three traditional forms of practice guidelines have in common is the fact that they typically evolved as reflections of "usual" practice. Their creation was mainly intuitive, growing out of the collective experience of mental health professionals and reflecting practices of these persons and their colleagues. Their existence was based on the tautology that what was done is what should be done and, by definition, whatever the "doctor" did was appropriate.

The written criteria sets were most often intended for use by payers and other sanctioning organizations. Table 1 contains examples of this type of criterion taken from the *Manual of Psychiatric Peer Review* (3rd Edition) of the American Psychiatric Association (1985).

The purpose of statements such as those in Table 1 was primarily to allow the identification of "outliers"—clinical episodes in which practice patterns appeared to be at significant variance from the norm, as defined by the criteria themselves. The terms "usual and customary" were ubiquitous among guidelines of this type. The guidelines themselves typically were written with a lack of specificity which virtually ensured that the definition of usual and customary subsumed a vast array of professional practices, all of which would be regarded as appropriate. As might be expected given that their development was intuitive and essentially *ad hoc,* these statements were only incidentally reflective of sound health care.

Regional Variations

A second characteristic shared by traditional guidelines is that they explicitly allowed for geographic variations in practice patterns. They commonly included qualifiers such as "depending upon local norms" and "as statistically determined by local guidelines". This meant, for example, that while a 28-day hospital stay for major depression might be accepted without question as reasonable in a city such as New York, it might be considered excessively long (and, hence, an "outlier") in Oklahoma City.

What accounted for such regional variations? Based on an empirical investigation of variations in medical care, Wennberg (1987) concluded that they were due primarily to providers' lack of knowledge about

Table 1

Model Screening Criteria Format for Adult Inpatient Treatment[1]

DIAGNOSES: *Major depression*
                    Depression with psychotic features
                    Dysthymic disorder

ADMISSION REVIEW

    A. *Reasons for Admission*

        1. Potential danger to self, others, or property, or

        2. Need for continuous skilled observation, high dose
           medication, or therapeutic milieu, and

        3. Impaired social, familial, or occupational
           functioning.

        4. Legally mandated admission

    B. *Initial Length of Stay Assignment*

    Locally established based on statistical norms.

CRITICAL DIAGNOSTIC AND THERAPEUTIC SERVICES

A.	Treatment plan to include problem formulation, treatment goals, and therapeutic modality (e.g., psychotherapy, pharmacotherapy, social therapies, behavior modification).	100%
B.	More than two psychotropic medications at any given time.	0%
C.	Change of psychotropic medications more than twice during any 7-day period.	0%
D.	ECT	0%

---

[1]APA, 1985, pp. 60-61

efficacy of alternative treatment strategies. Given the apparent significant effect of theoretical orientation on mental health practices, regional variations in mental health service patterns were probably also related to variations in the predominant theoretical orientation of service providers across regions.

It is critical to note that the regional variations reflected in such criteria sets were merely acknowledgments of actual variations observed in practice. At the same time, however, the long-standing tradition of accepting these variations gave a legitimacy to differences which frequently had no basis in science. The instrumental power of such standards was such as to consolidate them in third party reimbursement patterns.

The Movement Toward Accountability

Within the last decade, there has been a significant increase in the expectations of payers and purchasers of health services regarding accountability in professional services delivery. In the light of spiralling health care costs, large employers in particular have felt forced to participate as active players in the health care marketplace. In this new role, and armed with the capacity to self insure, these large purchasers are having significant influence, not only on the mechanisms for payment, but also on the actual patterns of service delivery. This new capacity to dictate is a striking departure from the traditional role of employers as passive purchasers. The more traditional third-party payers have also adopted a more assertive stance, partly in response to the demands from their corporate customers for more accountability.

One of the responses to the call for accountability has been an attempt to bring research findings on efficacy into practice to better ensure that what is done and paid for is what actually works. Other developments, increasingly obvious within the last decade, have combined with the pressures for increased accountability to create a fertile environment for the movement aimed at bringing research into mental health practice. Among these developments are:

1. *An improved ability of researchers and practitioners to be specific about treatment techniques and outcome.* In particular, researchers such as Aaron Beck (Beck, Hollon, Young et al., 1985) and Myrna Weissman (Weissman, Klerman, Prusoff et al., 1981) have made fundamental

contributions in the development of highly structured treatment strategies (Cognitive Therapy and Interpersonal Therapy, respectively) which have been formalized in manuals and subjected to careful evaluations of their efficacy. These researchers as well as others have provided excellent models for specifying the types of problems being treated, the types of changes being sought, and, most importantly, the specific procedures used to facilitate change.

2. *Increased federal government support for large scale, multi-site research programs aimed at specific treatment methods for specific problems such as depression and panic disorder.* This phenomenon alone has contributed significantly to the beginnings of a vastly improved data base reflecting a range of mental health and substance abuse problems. In recent years federal government support has been expanded to the actual development of medical practice guidelines (Goodwin, 1990).

3. *Increasing use of the computer in health care, resulting in improved access to information about problems, treatment strategies, and outcomes.* Access to relatively large data bases has enabled evaluators not only to make better estimates of efficacy of alternative treatments, but also to assess the utility and validity of emerging sets of practice guidelines.

4. *Increasing awareness among third party payers about mental health and substance abuse treatment.* As the emphasis on behavioral health services in the marketplace has increased, the traditionally physician-dominated insurance companies have come to realize the need for expertise specific to this specialty, and are increasing their in-house resources to deal with mental health and substance abuse issues. At the same time, the new, competing managed care specialty organizations—developed and controlled by experienced mental health professionals—are assuming a dominant position in the mental health market place. As a result of their increasing sophistication, these organizations are better able to assess both the problems of service delivery and potential solutions.

5. *An erosion of the general proscription on sharing of confidential patient information, partly as a result of payers' demands for accountability.* Without access to clinical information it would be impossible to "manage" care, let alone evaluate the utility and validity of guidelines used in its assessment. Mental health practitioners historically have maintained a firm commitment to yielding to the payer minimal clinical

information, and making any information which was submitted as innocuous as possible (Sharfstein, Towery, & Milowe, 1980). Provider behaviors, if not their attitudes, appear to be changing in the face of increasing demands for information combined with evidence that such information is generally used appropriately.

THE NEW PRACTICE GUIDELINES

Historically, the main role of practice policies has been to summarize usual practice. The role of newer guidelines is to summarize appropriate practice, defined as embodying intervention strategies shown by empirical research to be efficacious. Obviously, however, it remains necessary to supplement research findings with the consensus of expert judgment.

Eddy (1990b) provides a taxonomy for the methods which have been used for developing practice policies. The four types vary with respect to the relative contributions of professional judgment and analysis of research findings. The traditional method, which results in guidelines reflecting usual practice, is subsumed under the first type.

1. *Practice policies based on global subjective judgment.* This method includes, and is similar to, the traditional process of criterion development in that it relies primarily on the collective judgment of experts. Their judgment is informed by their own experiences and their knowledge of usual practice.

Under newer strategies the development of policies is systematic and strategic in contrast to the rather *ad hoc* and evolutionary process of the past.

2. *Evidence-based practice policies.* Under this method, groups of professionals still make judgments, but they do so after reviewing empirical research related to efficacy of various treatments. So, rather than being informed only by the personal experiences and knowledge of the judges, these judgments are informed additionally by scientific research.

3. *Outcomes-based practice policies.* Under this method the judges review the research literature as they do under the evidenced-based process. To this they add a review of studies which provide quantitative estimates of the relative benefits and harms of alternative treatment techniques. For example, in the development of criteria for the treatment of major depression, judges would review literature

dealing with both "cure rates" and side effects of electroconvulsive therapy (ECT) versus drug treatment combined with verbal therapy.
4. *Preference-based practice policies.* This methodology is similar to the outcomes-based strategy, but judges also consider information on patient preferences. In the example of major depression mentioned above, the judges would factor into their decision-making what the literature reveals about the attitudes of patients toward ECT and antidepressant medication.

In general, the limitations inherent in current research technology in mental health result in practice guidelines being, at best, evidence-based. With the exception of meta-analysis, very few analytic tools have been used to generate quantitative estimates of likelihood of outcomes in mental health, such as has been done for some types of medical/surgical procedures (Eddy, 1990a). Hence, the best current guidelines for mental health services are almost always developed via a formal review of the relevant research literature and a subsequent qualitative analysis of the findings based on the professional judgment of one or more experts.

Contrasting Old with New Guidelines: An Example

It is useful to compare a traditional criteria set for treatment of depression with modern practice guidelines. Under traditional criteria such as those illustrated in Table 1, appropriate services for a patient with depression are defined as "Critical Diagnostic and Therapeutic Services." Specifically, the four criteria specify those services which one would expect to observe (A), and those which one would not expect to observe (B, C, and D) in the treatment of a depressed patient. This example focuses on inpatient treatment.

The "100%" associated with Criterion A means that the conditions listed there should be observed for all patients admitted for treatment of major depression. According to this criterion, all patients must have a treatment plan. In addition, the criterion rather vaguely covers just about anything that is typically done in context of mental health inpatient services for depression. The 0% listed with Criteria B, C, and D indicates that one would not expect the typical treatment plan to be characterized by these conditions.

One characteristic common to such criteria is their innocuous nature: few mental health practitioners would dispute their appropriateness. At the same time, the criteria provide little basis for making useful discriminations for any but the most unusual practice patterns.

In contrast, evidence-based guidelines would reflect empirical evidence of efficacy of various types of treatment strategies for depression. For example, relatively recent multi-site studies of treatment of depression provide some evidence about the types of patients whose recovery may be longer lasting if their treatment includes antidepressant medication. One such type is the depressed patient who has had three or more previous episodes of the same illness (Kupfer & Frank, 1987). A standard reflecting this finding would state that for such a patient the treatment plan should give evidence that the provider has either prescribed medication or at least given consideration to the use of antidepressants (allowing, of course, for extenuating circumstances such as the patient's previous non-response to these types of medications or his/her unwillingness to take them).

A second standard might address the use of particular types of medications in combination. In particular, there is evidence that combining a tri-cyclic antidepressant (TCA) and an MAO inhibitor (MAOI) could result in a serious adverse physical reaction in patients (Richelson, 1989). So, while the earlier criterion (Table 1, Criterion B) would question the simultaneous use of more than two psychotropic medications, the new practice standard would question the simultaneous use of a TCA and an MAOI. If a reviewer in a managed care organization observed a case of recurrent depression in which the provider makes no mention of medication, or a case of simultaneous TCA and MAOI administration, he or she would be required to question the practitioner concerning the treatment plan.

How Guidelines are Implemented

As with traditional criteria, the new practice guidelines are used as "screens." The ultimate decision to approve reimbursement for a treatment plan which has characteristics at variance with one or more guidelines rests with a mental health professional employed by the managed care company who consults with the provider about issues raised by the guidelines. In the examples discussed above, the purpose of the consultation would include attention to a provider's reasons for not using or considering medication or for prescribing both a TCA and an MAOI.

In general, it is impossible to determine definitively the applicability of a particular standard to a particular patient. Practice policies are written for the most common problems and types of patient. Outcome studies generally focus on groups, not individuals, and innumerable patient and contextual variables may have an impact on the development of a treatment strategy and the individual patient's response to it. Even in the reporting of controlled clinical trails, measures of central tendency (such as the mean) are generally provided. What would be more useful would be measures such as percentage of individuals improving—or becoming worse—as a consequence of an intervention. Further, a determination of the probabilities of particular types of reactions to particular treatment strategies are far beyond the capabilities of current research technologies.

If used properly, then, these new practice guidelines neither prescribe nor provide "recipes" for treating individual patients or clients. As noted by Eddy (1990c), "tailoring a practice policy to fit an individual patient is the essence of clinical judgment" (p. 1840). The ultimate responsibility for determining the treatment strategy is vested in the service provider.

What practice guidelines do, in effect, is to require that a provider who wishes to deliver services which differ from what scientific evidence suggests would be effective provide a reasonable justification for his or her treatment plan. In the discussion about the variation from policy which subsequently ensues between the provider and the managed care organization, the provider is educated about the rationale for the policy. Just as importantly, the case manager obtains information which may provide evidence relevant to the adequacy of the particular guideline. It is the advisory nature of guidelines that leads to the use of the term guideline rather than a standard, a term frequently used in the literature.

Where Did Practice Guidelines Originate?

The earliest set of evidence-based mental health policies of which the authors are aware is the set of review criteria developed by the American Psychological Association in 1977 (Claiborn, Biskin, & Friedman, 1982) for the peer review program of the Civilian Health and Medical Program of the Uniformed Services (CHAMPUS). While the criteria were based in large part on the traditional professional consensus (formal national surveys of practice) and expert opinion, the Association also made a concerted effort to seek empirical support for criteria whenever possible. These early criteria, though modest efforts when compared to

the evidence-based sets of today, were a major advance over their prede-
cessors and were considered state-of-the-art in the late seventies.

Since that time the major thrust in the development of evidence-based
guidelines in mental health has been with private-sector, proprietary
managed care corporations. These corporations all report having their
own sets of empirically based guidelines.

Should Practice Policies Shape Practice?

In the late seventies, when managed care programs were in their infancy,
the major criticism of criteria used by those programs in the monitoring
of service delivery was that they would, in the words of the critics, "shape
practice" or "stifle innovation". The two major mental health professional associations, which at that time supported the dominant review
programs in mental health (Shueman & Penner, 1989), were especially
defensive in the presence of this criticism since it came from their own
constituents. The associations went to considerable lengths to educate
their members to the fact that criteria functioned only as screens and that
a final decision on payment for services was made only after a professional peer of the provider exercised his or her judgment to evaluate the
necessity and appropriateness of treatment. This explanation did not
mollify many, however, who appeared offended by the mere existence of
written criteria which defined appropriateness with any degree of
specificity.

To be "innovative" in providing services was represented by providers
as an almost sacred right of mental health practitioners. This stance was
somewhat ironic in view of the fact that the literature at that time
provided evidence for the existence of between 200 and 300 different
psychosocial therapies. The additional irony was that most providers,
rather than wishing to innovate, wanted to continue their "usual and
customary" practices, practices which had evolved over the course of
their careers as service providers.

The criticism about shaping practice or stifling innovation gives little
if any pause to those working in managed care today. The general belief
is that shaping practice is appropriate if the shaping process results in
services becoming safer and more effective. To the extent that Wennberg
(1987) is correct in his conclusion that variations in treatment have to do
with lack of knowledge among providers of services, it would seem
critical to impart to providers information about efficacy. The use of

evidence-based criteria would seem to be an excellent vehicle for doing this.

Misuse of Practice Guidelines

A number of forces serve to attenuate the professional development role of evidence-based practice criteria. These are dynamics which relate to the particular means by which the guidelines are applied and to their proprietary nature which, until recently, has kept them from being distributed to anyone outside of the case management company.

Problems in Application

While it is only reasonable to assert that current practice policies should function as guidelines and should be flexible at the point of individual application, in practice this has often not been the case. What is observed frequently within managed care organizations is misunderstanding of the appropriate use of practice guidelines by those responsible for implementing them—a misunderstanding mirrored in the provider community. Despite instruction to the contrary, case managers and reviewers frequently regard guidelines as immutable and may simply deny reimbursement for a service which is at variance with even a single criterion. One reason for this is inadequate training. Secondarily, the literal interpretation of guidelines often seems to result from a desire among these employees to streamline their work. Case managers and reviewers may have large numbers of cases to monitor (one industry standard, for example, is one case manager for every 25,000 covered lives) and, from their perspective, it is much more efficient to approve or deny a claim on the basis of discrete criteria than to discuss, negotiate, or call in a consultant.

These obvious explanations do not, however, adequately account for this problem. Written guidelines tend to be reified (if observed at all). While those who create practice guidelines are generally aware of their inadequacies (partly because of the difficulties experienced interpreting research studies), those who implement them tend to view them as immutable.

Problems with the Proprietary Nature of Guidelines

Existing practice guidelines have been developed almost exclusively in the private sector. As such they are proprietary and, until very recently,

have been considered trade secrets. Typically providers acquired knowledge of guidelines, if at all, in context of feedback about individual
treatment plans which were judged to violate one or more of those
guidelines. Under such circumstances, education of the provider was
haphazard at best, since feedback was both incomplete and non-systematic.
At the same time, providers often resented the secrecy, criticizing managed care companies for attempting to influence their practice patterns
without sharing with them the guidelines which describe what were
considered appropriate practices. Finally, this commitment to secrecy
meant that managed care companies as a group did not have the opportunity to share information essential to the continuous revision and improvement of guidelines.

This manifestation of the conflict between competitive advantage and
professional education was one of the unwelcome corollaries of privatized
health care. Fortunately, however, increasing numbers of the major managed mental health care companies now make their criteria sets available
to their network providers and, by extension, to the public. This change
seems to be largely related to the desire on the part of these companies to
ensure that the network providers who work for them identify with their
system. A criteria set is, after all, a clear statement of a philosophical
approach to treatment, and a lack of commitment to the approach on the
part of those who provide the services may limit the effectiveness of the
service system.

External versus Internal Sanctions

There are two major strategies for attempting to ensure quality within
a health care delivery system: external and internal. Under the external
strategy, monitoring systems are established which in various ways encourage or reward practitioners for providing services consistent with the
externally determined guidelines for quality (or punish them for failure
to do so). Under the internal strategy, practitioners themselves are involved
both in the development of the guidelines and in the process by which
the compliance of the particular provider community in this regard is
assured.

Managed care organizations vary in the extent to which they use
external versus internal strategies, but the prevailing approach is the
former. This is unfortunate in view of the consensus among experts in
quality assurance that, while external monitoring is a critical component
of any QA program, the optimal means to raise the technical quality of

care is through involvement of the service providers in development, implementation, and validation of practice policies. This sort of participation increases understanding of the rationale of guidelines and minimizes threats to provider acceptance. Providers require, in addition, access to educational and technical assistance to ensure that they have the knowledge and skills to comply with the new policies.

Lomas, Anderson, Domnick-Pierre et al. (1989) investigated the effect of widely disseminated practice guidelines on the actual practice of physicians. They found that, while a very large percentage of the practitioners knew about the guidelines and seemed to be predisposed to change practices to those recommended, dissemination of the guidelines resulted in only a slight change in actual practice. The authors concluded that practice policies

> ...should not be developed in isolation from other initiatives to modify inappropriate practice.... They do not appear likely to meet the ultimate objective of quality assurance with respect to changes in the behavior of physicians within a reasonable time, unless they are embedded in a broader program that addresses the need for translation and implementation of the guidelines locally (p. 1310).

This finding underscores the promise of the internal approach to guideline development. It is only with the participation and concurrence of providers in the development and review of guidelines that the managed system can expect their implementation to result in quality enhancement.

Neglecting the "Art" of Care

The practice guidelines discussed in this chapter focus exclusively on technical aspects of care. The "art" of care (see, for example, Donabedian, 1980) is neglected. This means that current systems of monitoring may increase the probability of service providers doing the "right" thing, but they cannot ensure that providers do it well. If one conceptualizes the professional armamentarium of mental health practitioners as consisting of attitude, knowledge, and skill competencies (Bent, 1986), it follows that the implementation of practice guidelines primarily involves knowledge competencies.

Some argue that influencing the attitudes and skills of mental health practitioners is not an appropriate concern of managed mental health programs. Such people believe, for example, that those providers who do not have the skills will be removed from managed systems due to poor outcomes. In contrast, there is at least one managed care organization which accepts only those provider applicants who participate in a formal retraining to ensure that they have the skills required to work within a managed care context.

CONCLUSION

One might reasonably assume that the impetus for the development and implementation of practice guidelines in mental health and chemical dependency would have come from three groups: (1) the professional training programs; (2) the academic/research community; and (3) the major professional associations. While the latter two groups have been active in the development of guidelines, all three have been conspicuously absent as direct sanctioners of their use.

The prime movers in the implementation of guidelines have been the managed care organizations. The knowledge-rich professional associations with their sophistication in theory-research-practice linkages not only have failed to support implementation of guidelines, but also have actively opposed them. The reasons are complex but are generally related to guild-oriented foci and political divisions within the organized disciplines, their opposition to anything but traditional fee-for-service payment systems, and their fear of litigation vis-à-vis restraint of trade and practice liability.

One prevailing characteristic of these professional disciplines has been their commitment to maintaining the mystification of their professional activities by resisting external demands for accountability. To endorse practice guidelines is to adopt a demystifying, consumerist stance.

That the providers and their professional associations should be active participants in the processes of development and implementation is highly desirable, but not crucial. Guidelines central to benefit design, utilization review, and case management are here to stay. Market forces require it. Nonetheless, one of the definitive challenges to managed care is its capacity eventually to embrace a change in forms for practice guidelines from a cost containment to a true quality enhancement role. This is a system change of large magnitude and will require the input of many groups in a context of reasoned collegial, interdisciplinary debate and problem solving.

REFERENCES

American Psychiatric Association. (1985). *Manual of Psychiatric Peer Review* (3rd Edition). Washington, D.C.: Author.

Beck, A.T., Hollon, S.D., Young, J.E., et al. (1985). Treatment of depression with cognitive therapy and amitriptyline. *Archives of General Psychiatry, 42,* 142–148.

Bent, R.J. (1986). Toward quality assurance in the education of practicing psychologists. In J.E. Callan, D.R. Peterson, & G. Stricker, *Quality in Professional Psychology Training: A National Conference and Self-Study.* National Council of Schools of Professional Psychology, 27–36.

Berwick, D.M. (1989). Continuous improvement as an ideal in health care. *New England Journal of Medicine, 320,* 53–56.

Claiborn, W.L., Biskin, B.H., & Friedman, L.S. (1982). CHAMPUS and quality assurance. *Professional Psychology, 13,* 40–49.

Donabedian, A. (1980). *Explorations in Quality Assessment and Monitoring:* Vol. 1. *The Definition of Quality and Approaches to its Assessment.* Ann Arbor, MI: Health Administration Press.

Eddy, D. (1990a). Anatomy of a decision. *Journal of the American Medical Association, 263,* 441–443.

Eddy, D. (1990b). Practice policies: Guidelines for methods. *Journal of the American Medical Association, 263,* 1839–1841.

Eddy, D. (1990c). Practice policies: What are they? *Journal of the American Medical Association, 263,* 877–880.

Eddy, D. (1990d). Practice policies: Where do they come from? *Journal of the American Medical Association, 263,* 1265–1275.

Goodwin, F. (1990). Keeping the behavioral health care industry accountable to patients and their families. Behavioral Healthcare Tomorrow Conference, San Francisco, September 15, 1990.

Kupfer, D.J. & Frank, E. (1987). Relapse in recurrent unipolar depression. *American Journal of Psychiatry, 144,* 86–88.

Lomas, J., Anderson, G.M., Domnick-Pierre, K., et al (1989). Do practice guidelines guide practice? *Journal of the American Medical Association, 321,* 1306–1311.

Richelson, E. (1989). Antidepressants: Pharmacology and clinical use. In American Psychiatric Association Task Force on Treatments of Psychiatric Disorders, *Treatments of Psychiatric Disorders.* Washington, D.C.: American Psychiatric Association, 1773–1786.

Sharfstein, S.S., Towery, O.B., & Milowe, I.D. (1980). Accuracy of diagnostic information submitted to an insurance company. *American Journal of Psychiatry, 137,* 70–73.

Shueman, S.A. & Penner, N.R. (1988). Administering a national program of mental health peer review. In G. Stricker & A.R. Rodriguez (Eds.), *Handbook of Quality Assurance in Mental Health.* New York: Plenum, 441–454.

Weissman, M.M., Klerman, G.L., Prusoff, B.A., et al (1981). Depressed outpatients:

Results one year after treatment with drugs and/or interpersonal psychotherapy. *Archives of General Psychiatry, 38,* 51–55.

Wennberg, J.E. (1987). Paradox of appropriate care. *Journal of the American Medical Association, 258,* 2568–2569.

PART V
EDUCATION, TRAINING, AND PROVIDER DEVELOPMENT

PART V: INTRODUCTORY NOTE

The introduction of managed care programs has brought to light a significant number of system problems affecting behavioral health services. These include problems with the financing system, education and training, professional socialization, and legislation and regulation. The problems in professional training are particularly vexing, at least in part because the academic foundations of professional training programs make change in response to external demands particularly unlikely. In Chapter 10, Troy proposes that the solutions to the problems affecting the quality of behavioral health services can only come from a collaborative effort of professional training programs and the managed care industry.

A major thesis of this chapter on developing competencies among mental health professionals is that most training programs do not have among their faculty the expertise needed to treat the critical issues of managed care. Furthermore, their commitment to a core set of knowledge and skills precludes significant expansion of the curriculum to embrace issues of managed care. Finally, specialization in clinical practice is generally considered to be in the realm of post-graduate training.

It would seem, therefore, that managed care companies will need to take a leadership role with regard to professional training. This will require collaborative efforts with training programs to develop formal practicum, internship, and post-doctoral training experiences for students of those programs. It will also require the managed care programs themselves, perhaps in consultation with training programs, to develop strategies for retraining of practicing mental health professionals according to the needs of managed systems.

Chapter 10

DEVELOPING AND IMPROVING
PROFESSIONAL COMPETENCIES

WARWICK G. TROY

Advocacy and lobbying efforts by the major mental health professional associations aimed at the sanctioners of health care services have consistently and relentlessly proclaimed that mental health services are an integral and critical part of general health care. Advocates have identified the contribution of behavioral science applications to health services provision in the form of enhanced health outcomes. This lobbying has been met with signal success.

One of the problematic consequences of this effort, however, has been the guild-oriented argument for *general* psychotherapy as a health services intervention of manifest efficacy. This claim is both undiscriminating and self-serving. The case for the efficacy of non-focused, non-strategic, longer term, dynamic or eclectic psychotherapy provided by independent practitioners working in disciplinary and organizational isolation, without the benefit of practice standards or guidelines, empirically derived intervention protocols, a quality management context, or the framework of a differentiated system of services provision, is marginal at best.

When "psychotherapy" is demonstrated to be efficacious it is invariably associated with the very contingencies whose prevailing absence has just been noted in most circumstances surrounding the actual provision of most psychotherapy. Claiming that psychotherapy is, per se, an integral part of the full complement of health services provision does not make it so; nor does claiming that psychotherapists can be readied appropriately for the field of managed behavioral health by some additional exposure to brief therapy in their graduate training together with an induction program on entering the context of managed care.

This issue in many ways encapsulates the challenge to professional education and training, to the provider community, to the professional associations, and to the managed care industry itself: effective behavioral health providers in managed care are made, not born. Trite though the observation may appear, far too great a proportion of the membership of the above communities would appear not to have heard it. As shall become clear, the lamentable state of professional education and training in general, and with respect to managed care in particular, attests to the fact that these key stakeholder groups have much to answer for.

How should blame for these distortions be apportioned among these stakeholder communities?

- To the *professional education community* for not having seriously attempted to prepare graduate students for the world of practice, let alone managed care.
- To the *professional associations* whose self-serving guild interests let them continue to wink at the manifest deficiencies of professional training programs and the unacceptably low levels of professional competencies within the provider community; for their pusillani- mous attitude toward standards of practice implementation and the development of appropriate mechanisms for quality management; for their sustained, active resistance to the inexorable growth of managed care; and for their unexamined public espousal of the merits of generic psychotherapy as a health services intervention.
- To the *provider community* for its minimalist concern with practic- ing beyond one's competence and with acquisition of appropriate competencies through continuing education; for its general aban- donment of organized care settings and the public sector care ethic; and for its reluctance to be held accountable to consumers, payers and sanctioners.
- To the *managed care industry* for its propensity for competing on price, not quality; for being indiscriminate in its selection of providers; for an undeveloped commitment to on-the-job training and professional development for providers and case managers; and for clumsy, alienating case management processes.

What is Wrong with the World of Professional Practice, Training, and the Managed Care Industry?

The second managed care revolution is upon us—with a vengeance— and the world of professional education and training is poorly prepared for the nature, magnitude, and urgency of the task ahead. The world of practice must change and must do so rapidly, in order merely to survive. There is an urgency, markedly lacking even two years ago, and it places a premium on practitioners who possess a discrete armamentarium of competencies supported by appropriate attitudes and values embracing consumer diversity and traditionally underserved groups (Graham & Fox, 1991).

The formal, university-based training programs—always unrepentantly behind—are now further behind than ever. At the same time, entrepreneurial training organizations are springing up and offering "cookbook," essentially atheoretical approaches to retraining, oblivious to the requirements of appropriate instructional design or the wider context of industry needs.

It is problematic but true that effective service standards have not been promulgated or supported by mental health professional associations. In their preoccupation with avoiding legal exposure, the guilds will find that the world has also passed them by. Business speculation, economic entrepreneurism, and a strong sense that anything is possible are driving the health service industry. It is too late to lament, as many professionals do, that managed care is preoccupied with cost containment (it is); that managed care is concerned less with managing than with rationing (true); that providers are inadequately involved in benefit plan design (true); or that managed care companies are more concerned with the immediate imperatives of surviving competition than longer term investment in formal evaluation of services provision (true).

The chaos which now exists has both structural and normative components. And, indeed, there is a great deal wrong with how managed care companies operate. At the same time, there is much that is promising, and it is these promising aspects which must be identified and promoted to ensure they are retained in future revisions of managed systems and their support infrastructures.

What Resources Do We Possess That Can Be Used To Fix Things?

There is much in the current service environment to cause optimism about the future of behavioral health care. For example:

- *We know a lot about managed care.* The sine qua non of managed care is a staff or group model prepaid plan—the HMO. HMOs have been going on quietly for over half a century. In many ways they are models of accountability. Although their record in health care, and in particular mental health and chemical dependency, is not perfect, these long standing organizations must be taken as exemplars in a field where variations in quality threaten the viability of the industry. Providing services of high quality in a managed context is not beyond current capabilities. The successful model we are familiar with is traditional large, public, organized care settings using salaried clinicians. The challenge will be to translate these accomplishments within the current private, entrepreneurial climate.

- *We know a lot about service planning and organization.* Available technology includes health status, clinical process, and services outcome measures; management information systems; utilization review and provider and consumer profiling techniques; and procedures for estimating service costs.
- *We have access to useful public health concepts.* Mental health has traditionally made little use of public health concepts, but in the new health care environment, their application to mental health and chemical dependency is more obvious. These concepts include population-based approaches, the composition of a comprehensive set of services and their functional integration, case management and continuity of care, primary prevention and early intervention approaches to at-risk groups, the concepts of wellness and health promotion, the nature of chronicity, and a technology of enablement rather than disability.
- *We have a range of proven intervention techniques.* Commonly used and reliable interventions targeted to meet the needs of the consumer and service system rather than the expectations of the provider include developmental, whole-of-life approaches to services provision; the strategic use of information; self help and psycho-educational approaches; and targeted systems interventions involving client, family, carers, and other potential resources. Such strategies are efficacious and serve to demystify behavioral health services provision. They are consumer friendly and empower the client.

Effective exploitation of the resources require, however, that we acknowledge what is unstable as well as insubstantial in the present context of behavioral health care.

Chaotic Nature of the Industry

The severity of the problems besetting graduate professional training can not be minimized by observations that professional training in the health sciences and, indeed, generically, is inherently incapable of truly effective strategic preparation for practice. The situation is particularly serious because the world of training is increasingly out of touch with practice, and because the managed behavioral health care industry is currently extremely unstable.

Any measured view of the industry reveals a multiform and ever-changing world. Managed behavioral health care is represented by a wide variety of formal administrative arrangements. Variation abounds in the areas of financing and reimbursement systems; in disciplinary groupings of providers; in the structures and processes of services provision; in services monitoring; in ways in which providers are recruited, selected, monitored, and supported; and in the inconsistent and *ad hoc* nature of quality assessment and management. If the proliferation of managed care companies and the disturbingly high prevalence of individual providers being associated with multiple plans are added to this depiction, the chaos seems self-evident.

A Commitment to Quality as a Response to Instability within the Industry

In practice, the atheoretic and utilitarian nature of managed systems give cause to sceptics to doubt the capacity of the organizations to develop and deliver services that are accessible, appropriate, efficacious, and cost-effective (VandenBos, 1993; Sharfstein, 1992). Such doubts will legitimately invoke questions about the quality of managed behavioral health services in the absence of an explicit and measured industry-wide focus on quality assessment and management.

Absent an effective role for education and training programs in professional competency development for providers, it will be very difficult for the managed care industry to realize the goal of consistently high-quality services. This is by no means to say, however, that a "return of the academy to the world of practice," no matter how well conceived and articulated, will alone be sufficient to attain the quality management goal. The industry itself must assume a significant responsibility for such an enterprise. A true partnership between the academic/professional training community and the managed behavioral health care industry must develop (Blackwell & Schmidt, 1992).

The involvement of the training community is a necessary, but not a sufficient, condition to establish some kind of structure within the chaos so endemic to the industry. It is appropriate that this structure be raised on the principles and mechanisms of quality in health services, and that a functional partnership be a prime vehicle by which it can develop and endure.

The next section examines the kinds of generic competencies that are to be developed in the trained clinician which at once serve the tenets of quality in service provision and meet the industry's requirements for competent and well-trained clinicians.

Generic Competency Development

It must be emphasized that the pre-doctoral professional training program is, *sui generis*, overcrowded. The pressures to expand the curriculum, to become more "relevant", to provide for the mastery of yet another skill or knowledge base are unrelenting. Pressure to particularize the curriculum must, however, be resisted. This will to resist is critical for reasons other than the essential ungovernability and lack of consumer acceptance of a training curriculum inflated in content and duration. What must eventually emerge, nonetheless, is a professional training climate less hostile to market forces and structures, and capable of a more anticipatory role in mental and behavioral health. In turn, this more open climate will yield a curriculum incorporating two significant reforms. The first of these is a multifaceted and integrated curriculum with clear focus on the development of an irreducible set of professional competencies, embracing the knowledge, skills, and attitudes/values appropriate to the changing world of practice (Bent, 1986).

A competency-based curriculum must, however, be able to do more than provide a sound base for the developing practitioner to engage in a complex professional world. The curriculum must also provide the kind of framework which will enable the trainee not merely to cope with, but also to anticipate and reframe, his or her professional world. This is the second of the key proposed curricular reforms: the capacity of new training programs to induce mastery of competencies of substantial conceptual depth and complexity to facilitate effective coping with subsequent unfamiliar inputs. This is the essence of a generic approach to training and one based upon what David Ausubel, over 30 years ago, termed "advance organizers"—the deep conceptual underpinnings of the program. Such an approach counters the prevailing mode of *ad hoc* expansion of content, skill by skill and fact by fact, within a distended and poorly integrated curriculum.

The development, implementation, and monitoring of a training curriculum yielding a discrete set of competencies with considerable generalizability are, collectively, the signal challenge to pre-doctoral and postdoctoral professional training programs. Their success in doing this, together with the effectiveness of whatever partnership the programs can forge with the behavioral health managed care industry, will largely determine whether academe will continue to be marginalized at the edge of practice or whether the education and training community can begin to put its stamp on the changing world of behavioral health practice (see Hoshmand & Polkinghorne, 1992).

The responsibility for the development of competencies appropriate to the professional role of providers in managed care can not, at this stage, be restricted to pre-doctoral education and training programs. The managed care industry itself must play a major and direct role now and into the foreseeable future.

What Kind of World will Professional Training Need to Anticipate?

Despite real chaos and a distinctly problematic context of care, it is both appropriate and realistic to emphasize those resources which have served the field well and will continue to do so. The situation would be greatly improved if services were provided through systems, similar to HMOs, which were capitated and responsible for the delivery of an essential packet of care. Such organizations would be staffed with providers having a service ethos similar to that of providers in public organized care settings, such as the CMHCs of 20 years ago. In addition, they would (1) actively promote the use of available technology, (2) apply key principles of population-based public health approaches in services planning and delivery; (3) re-emphasize developmental and educational service techniques, and (4) actually begin to use the rich corpus of information which provides a true technology for services development, implementation, and evaluation.

Creating effective systems requires both a recapturing of what is known to be efficacious and a dedication to the use of mechanisms to better advance quality and accountability. Such an approach is consumer-oriented and, therefore, needs-based and outcomes driven. It is flexible and involves and empowers the consumer in a collaborative endeavor. It is systems-oriented. It is prevention focused and is as much concerned with minimizing exposure to risk as with appropriate remediation. Accordingly, it acknowledges and directly confronts the challenges of human diversity. It values what science and technology can offer, while acknowledging the shortcomings of exclusively positivist approaches. It is manifestly not designed for the provider, yet it welcomes the provider as an essential collaborator, and values the provider as both a clinician and a repository for a science of practice (Hoshmand & Polkinghorne, 1992). It is not guild-oriented, yet it offers a partnership with learned societies, institutions, and professional associations in issues affecting quality of care, training, services development, and applied research.

Systems require institutional frameworks. In turn, these require providers and service managers linked by a shared normative stance, working in teams in cooperative modes, deriving from many disciplines, working in a professional climate with clear and differentiated professional roles, guided by an unambiguous set of policies and procedures which affect their clinical input and denote clear levels of operational responsibility. It is a system in which staff understand and welcome the concept of financial risk, understand health financing arrangements and capitation, and are committed to the discharge of formal accountability obligations, both professional and public.

To construct such a system on a far larger scale than has hitherto been the case is, of course, the challenge. It requires providers to assume new roles, acquire new skills and knowledge, and adopt new attitudes. The education, training, and professional development of clinicians requires not only an explicit training/development focus, but also a structure and a mechanism.

What Kind of Provider does the Industry Require?

It is somewhat paradoxical that the competencies required by the industry of its providers are such as ought to be immediately available within any cohort of graduate clinicians. The particular set of such competencies which would serve the industry well is hardly arcane; nor is it difficult to conceive of. Yet much has been made of the functional chasm between the new graduate's limited professional armamentarium and the kinds of knowledge, attitudes and skills that will be required of him or her in the world of managed care (Belar, 1989; Blackwell &

Schmidt, 1992; Boaz, 1988; VandenBos, 1993). That there is such a gap is to be explained more by deficiencies in graduate training than by either the arcane nature or complexity of the tasks which confront the provider in managed behavioral health care.

What the industry does require is, first, that providers have a well developed and articulated set of attitudes and values relating to *professional responsibility:* that is, they are comfortable in being held accountable for their work and they freely participate in activities which are associated with the mechanisms of accountability, such as peer review, outcome-oriented research, and provider profiling. Second, the industry expects that providers are knowledgeable of and comfortable with working within the *constraints of a large system* in which many kinds of interdependencies are manifest: among one's professional colleagues, between providers and case reviewers and administrators, and between service subsystems. Third, the industry would expect a general awareness of the mechanisms associated with *integration and continuity of care,* particularly within a "closed" system such as the traditional, prepaid plans (Belar, 1989). Fourth, it would expect the provider to possess competence in both the development of individualized service plans and *clinical documentation.* Finally, managed care would require of the provider a *varied mix of intervention skills* together with the capacity to employ these skills with flexibility and precision.

These "requirements" or "expectations" are by no means unique to managed care. Neither are they new. But for the fragmentation of health services provision, the traditional autonomy of the provider and the lack of accountability attendant upon such a status, the over-inclusive identification of mental health services with psychotherapy, the enshrinement of the independent practitioner, the neglect of the public care system, the absence of any clearly articulated national mental health policy (Kiesler, 1992), and the remoteness of professional training from the world of practice—it might reasonably have been assumed that there would have been providers in abundance easily capable of meeting these modest expectations. For modest they are: they represent nothing more than an irreducible core of professional roles to be expected of any developed professional. And as for not being new, this set of five broad competencies has characterized the professional roles of mental health professionals in community mental health centers and, particularly, in HMOs for many decades. These roles are essentially those of providers who work effectively in organized care settings.

What the rapid growth of the managed care industry has done, therefore, is to re-identify a set of competencies that were once rather routine— competencies associated with service *systems* where professional *staff* communicate directly with each other about clients' needs and services; where individual clients have their care "case managed" to ensure that they do not "fall between the cracks," where senior staff serve as effective professional exemplars and preceptors for less experienced clinicians; and where mental health professionals routinely consult with, or are consulted by, medical, nursing, and allied health colleagues.

Let it at once be said, however, that such a commentary is designed neither to invoke a morally superior past, nor to claim that all is lost in the present. Just as there were all too many deficiencies in the community mental health centers, mental health providers in independent practice have made, collectively, a uniquely valuable contribution to mental health care in the U.S. The point of the commentary is in fact to re-assert that not only have mental health service delivery and the professions lost their way in the past 20 years, so too has the professional educational and training system. The former got it wrong with a laissez-faire, non-system, private sector response to mental health service provision, driven by for-profit corporations. The mental health professions for far too long promulgated only psychotherapy as the instrumental arm of behavioral health practice. The academy failed to discharge its responsibility for innovation by its inordinate focus on non-applied research, its exclusive emphasis on formalized clinical assessment and ideologically driven therapeutic "orientations" as a substitute for professional training, and a remoteness from practitioners and organized care settings.

Approaches to Curricular Reform in Professional Education and Training

What the development of managed care models has achieved, then, is to force a reappraisal of how mental health care should be planned and provided, and to promote debate on what is deemed to be the irreducible core of good quality practice. As it improves, managed care will inevitably induce, and consume, those professional competencies most directly associated with developed systems of care. We have already considered what more enlightened services systems might look like. Reform of education and training must be directed at the acquisition of those competencies most directly associated with system interdependencies.

A number of authors has called, variously, for graduate and post-doctoral training to provide more directly and more appropriately for the current and emerging world of practice (Belar, 1989; Belar & Perry, 1992; Blackwell & Schmidt, 1992; Clements, 1992; Graham & Fox, 1992). Blackwell and Schmidt seek to have managed care organizations and educational institutions share responsibility for "defining and supporting training in managed mental health care" (p. 964). Most writers, however, limit the scope of reform either to the provision of additional discrete curricular offerings within the graduate curriculum, for example, legal liability (Applebaum, 1993; Monahan, 1993) and management skills (Clements, 1992), or to the modification of existing curricular offerings, such as short-term focussed psychotherapy (Austad et al., 1992; Belar, 1989; Blackwell & Schmidt, 1992; Boaz, 1988). VandenBos (1993), in invoking public health concepts such as primary care, usefully identifies a continuum of care for behavioral health services from preventive care through screening/early intervention to long-term care and rehabilitation as a desideratum for treatment planning within managed care.

Interestingly, Hoshmand and Polkinghorne's (1992) important analysis of the need for a mutuality of science and practice, which would allow practitioners to contribute to the knowledge base, does not mention the potential for managed care to facilitate such a rapprochement. Again, the report on the National Conference on Scientist-Practitioner Education and Training for the Professional Practice of Psychology (Belar & Perry, 1992) in discussing the experiential core of professional practice, also fails to acknowledge managed care systems, as do Graham and Fox (1992) in their call for "centers of excellence"—research and practice institutions to combat the disabling consequences of social and economic disruption for traditionally under served populations.

Curricular Content Appropriate to Managed Systems

Displayed in Table 1 are examples of professional competencies that are deemed relevant to behavioral health services under managed systems of care. For each of these broad competencies (column 1) is listed a set of content issues designed to illuminate the competency-in-practice and to be treated within a professional training curriculum (column 2). These latter content issues represent a distillation of the views of experts.

The value of such a representation is that it is fairly exhaustive. What this display does not do, however, is to distinguish among the content areas of column 2 the particular educational level (e.g., graduate or

Table 1

Curricular Examples of Behavioral Health Competencies for Managed Systems

Core Competencies	Examples of Curricular Content
1. Respect for Accountability to Consumers	1. Communication with client advocate Patient satisfaction Role of information resouces
2. Interventions	2. Short-term, focal, strategic Extended assessment Focus on system concepts More effective modalities Psycho-educational approaches Use of timely, appropriate information: self management
3. Care Planning/Case Management	3. Cost realities; impact of payment systems Interdisciplinary consultation Assessing client needs Use of collateral contacts
4. Continuity of Care	4. Prevention/early intervention Assessment Short- and medium-term treatment Episodic treatment Long-term rehabilitation Alternative service formats
5. Human Diversity	5. Individual differences Cultural and racial-ethnic differences Prevention
6. Socialization/Professional Roles	6. Communication/interprofessional linkages Interdisciplinary respect Cooperative working modes Collegial peer consultation Mthodology of clinical practice Provider profiling
7. Training/Supervision	7. Supervision/training/evaluation/feedback Training the trainer Interdisciplinary nexus

8. Ethics/Legal Issues	8. Facilitation of ethical decision process in
	    clinical work
	Legal responsibilities to review, disclose,
	    appeal, continue treatment
	Provider selection issues
	Risk management procedures, training

9. Administration/Management/Managed Care Systems	9. Resource utilization Mores/procedures of organization Organizational policy Ensuring access to services Smooth interface Continuity of care Rationing/queuing Health system design/population focus Benefit design

(Table 1 Continued)

10. The Health System	10. Health policy Health services organization Health services financing
11. Public Health Concepts	11. Population (catchment) focus Health status/at-risk groups Wellness, health promotion Continuity of care
12. Program Development	12. Development of educational programs
13. Research/Evaluation	13. Measuring the clinical process/outcomes Outcomes research Involving stakeholders in research/evaluation Utilization of research findings
14. Quality Assessment/Assurance	14. Defining quality Defining quality measures Involving stakeholders in QA Utilization of quality assessment findings

post-graduate) at which the issue should be treated within a training curriculum. Again, obviously, no distinction is made between what issues may be more profitably dealt with via local, inservice professional development formats and those that are better treated in more formal continuing education settings.

A final issue needs to be clarified regarding Table 1. In a previous section, five general expectations or "requirements" of providers associated with managed systems were identified. Clearly, the core competencies listed in column 1 of Table 1 do not appear to have much in common with the five "requirements" which managed behavioral health systems expect to see in providers working with them. This general lack of correspondence is due to the fact that the five desiderata are really best viewed as professional roles, or constellations of competencies. Put differently, they are global ways of conducting oneself as a professional provider. One may assume that a provider who satisfies the five "requirements" would have acquired some developed proficiency in each core competency in column 1.

Lastly, in considering Table 1, it should be emphasized that the curricular treatment of content issues listed in column 2 is not restricted to classroom settings. Such formats as supervised field-based training, individual and group supervision, contact with professional exemplars, empirical and action-research experience, community consultation, advocacy, and self-initiated professional development activities are educational modalities with an equal claim as vehicles of competency acquisition. Indeed, the cumulative effect of sequential exposure to these different modalities plays a critical, if poorly understood, role in the acquisition of the concepts which underpin competencies.

Confronting the Realities of Reform in Training

Reform programs must address issues such as the particular target group for which training is designed; the constraints and limitations of training (particularly graduate training); and the selection of operational strategies for the implementation of reform.

Where Will this Training Occur?

The development of professional competencies, vis-à-vis managed behavioral health care would seem to be restricted to three kinds of learning environments: (a) generic graduate education and training programs which would seek, in part, to anticipate the world of managed behavioral health; (b) more specific post-doctoral continuing education programs focusing on skill development deemed relevant to managed behavioral health (these could originate from within and without the industry); and (c) highly specific in-house, industry-based induction and provider development training programs designed and implemented by individual managed care companies. Of these three approaches, only the third, company-specific programs, escapes the obligation of dealing with the kind of variation in the managed care industry noted earlier in this chapter. For pre-doctoral education and training, the challenge is, as we have seen, the greatest. Nonetheless, the enduring viability of the managed behavioral health care industry and, more importantly, that of its consumers, depends very significantly upon all three approaches and the extent to which the potential of their differential contributions is realized.

Constraints on Graduate Training

Despite the emphasis thus far on the need for graduate training programs to anticipate the changed world of practice, it must be acknowledged that not only are there very real limits as to the capacity of training programs thus to prepare practitioners, but also to focus extensively on today's world of practice is to miss the target as this world inevitably changes.

There is, however, another reason why an inadequate preoccupation with the specifics of the present (however remote a possibility that may be for the academy) actually precludes the acquisition of an appropriate professional armamentarium. Effective educational design endeavors to create curricular content and learning formats which emphasize the acquisition of extremely general concepts: the broad principles involved in learning "how" as well as learning "what." Absent the acquisition of a limited number of key, overarching concepts of sufficient generality to guide professional decision making, professional education and training becomes little more than a large collection of recipes, each having to be learned in the particular; absent such concepts there is also no possibility of learning how to learn, of self-directed learning.

Training is at liberty to focus on specifics; education has a wider ambit. The graduate training program embraces both foci.

The primary task of graduate professional training is the education and training of a person who knows truly what it is to be a professional; who thinks, acts, and feels as a professional. This task transcends particular professions, and is facilitated through a large number of complex mechanisms, formal and informal, and many only incompletely documented. Yet this process of professional socialization, however generic its mechanisms, is mediated via exposure to a profession-specific content within a context also profession-specific. Thus it is pedagogically legitimate to observe that a graduate program in (for example) psychology seeks to develop multi-faceted professionals through exposure to the specialty field of clinical psychology. The point here is that socialization in the clinical psychology specialty area may be seen as the means to an end: an end which is, presumably, the production of a caring, competent, effective, and ethical clinical and behavioral scientist.

The prime objective for the education and training of behavioral health practitioners is the development of the generalist professional who possesses an array of generic competencies adequate to a wide variety of applications—across presenting problems, modes of intervention, and service formats. The same person is, however, also expected to demonstrate competencies generalizable to research, teaching, consultation, and the like. Lastly, as we have discussed at length, this individual is now also expected to be able to function with fluency and competence in the unfamiliar world of managed care. How may these apparently competing requirements be realized within a unitary specialty professional training program?

Let us consider the following three propositions about graduate education and managed behavioral health care:

Proposition 1: One of the most efficacious approaches a graduate program can take regarding training for managed care is to develop entry-level clinicians possessing the kind of generic scientific and clinical competencies discussed above.

Proposition 2: The competencies required of the behavioral health practitioner under managed care are essentially those with which graduate training programs should always have been primarily concerned.

Proposition 3: The context of managed behavioral health care effectively illuminates those discrete sets of competencies which define an effective professional, both scientifically and clinically.

These propositions overlap considerably in terms of their general message; their foci are, however, different. Proposition 1, in speaking to graduate training programs, says, in essence: Don't be too concerned about the world of managed care; simply focus on preparing your entry-level professionals with a set of generic competencies. Your entry-level practitioners will then be prepared for anything. Proposition 2, in speaking to graduate training programs, says something very similar but appears to take the programs to task for not having known something (something they probably could not have known). Proposition 3 simply enjoins us detachedly to observe the world of managed behavioral health care. Were we to have done so properly we would, presumably, have recognized what constitutes a true professional.

The purpose of this exercise is twofold: first to make an unambiguous value statement about the primacy of generic professional competencies; second to argue strongly against those commentators who have tended to see the solution for graduate training programs vis-à-vis preparation for managed care as one involving modest tinkering with the existing curriculum together with a small increase in course offerings designed to introduce the trainee to managed care. Hoshmand and Polkinghorne (1992) are clearly correct: nothing less than an eventual wholesale restructuring of professional training will be adequate to meet the challenge.

Implementation Strategies for the Reform of Training

In the shorter term it is probably unrealistic to expect that many pre-doctoral training programs will be able to transcend their prevailing professional culture and limited resources sufficiently for them to effectively shape the competencies of developing providers vis-à-vis managed care. That said, there would seem some useful approaches academe could engage in.

Training programs should, first of all, explicitly and positively acknowledge the importance of the industry for the professional futures of graduate training and its products. This could set the stage for a true educational partnership between training programs and service systems. Second, training programs should establish formal training linkages at practicum, internship, and postdoctoral/residency levels with organized care settings connected with managed care companies, together with a commitment to exploit in a positive way these linkages for the purposes of behavioral health services research. This not only would meet an essential imperative for specialty accreditation for training programs—by ensuring the integration of theory, research, and practice—but also would provide managed care companies with much needed research capacity in both clinical outcomes management and services utilization.

Third, clinical training programs might consider a human resource sharing partnership in which trainees, particularly post-doctoral, would serve as administrative fellows in the managed care companies, while experienced behavioral health practitioners could be appointed to an academic team as adjunct members of the clinical faculty. Finally, in due course, the pre-doctoral training curriculum itself could come to embody some issues central to managed behavioral health care, such as quality assessment and management, prevention and health promotion, and mental health/behavioral health policy and financing.

There is, of course, little in these proposals which is not already an established part of the training fabric in the clinical health sciences, organization sciences, law, and business. The traditional scientific/research emphasis of the pre-doctoral training curriculum in professional psychology, however, has in indirect ways made the identification and implementation of the quite pedestrian *practice* linkages suggested above more difficult than it has been for other professional programs in health, law, and business. Indeed, it is interesting to note that a recent debate in the *Harvard Business Review* (November/December 1992) saw the industry (i.e., the world of business) taking the graduate business training programs to task for an over-emphasis on empirical research, lack of relevance to practice and management, and inadequate linkages with corporations. The world of behavioral health care has not, apparently, witnessed such public dissatisfaction with graduate training programs in its field. One wonders why.

Conclusion

Creating education and training environments appropriate to the rapidly changing world of health services, organization, and financing is a significant challenge for all health professions. Behavioral health providers have not, by and large, been well served by graduate training programs which have continued to be all too remote from the world of practice. Equity—and market-driven initiatives in health care organization and financing now make it imperative that graduate training programs and managed behavioral health care companies begin to forge functional partnerships to produce practitioners who possess a mix of generic competencies appropriate to the changed world. Unions of this kind must also confront the need for competency enhancement and retraining of providers associated with managed behavioral health networks as well as new inductees.

In order not to become utterly marginalized, graduate training programs need to develop training curricula which reflect not only a new armamentarium of applied behavioral science interventions, but a *radically altered conception of professional roles for the emerging practitioner.* Central to this is a set of attitude and value imperatives emphasizing accountability to consumers, payers, and sanctioners of health care. In addition, the developing practitioner will be exposed to a set of issues relating to health policy, financing, organization, and administration. Public health tenets such as continuity of care, primary prevention and health promotion, early identification of at-risk groups, together with basic epidemiological concepts will ultimately be formalized within these new "accountable" training curricula. So will familiarity with quality assessment mechanisms and quality management strategies. Knowledge of and sensitivity to the health needs of traditionally disadvantaged groups such as racial/ethnic minorities and children will be regarded as critical.

In short, the new mental health and chemical dependency provider will be prepared for and required to serve as a collegial, responsive, accountable, multi-skilled health services professional. Currently, the vast majority of graduate training programs possess neither the faculty mix nor the technological and management expertise to develop such programs. Nor, by and large, do they possess the kind of vision or institutional leadership essential to drive forward large scale innovation of this kind. It would seem that, for the more immediate future, a significant portion of the responsibility for provider development will have to be assumed by the managed care companies themselves. This industry-based training and development responsibility must initially concentrate on skill enhancement and a refocusing of the professional role of providers appropriate to the world of managed care.

The industry itself, training programs, providers, and consumers all stand to gain much from the development of partnerships between managed care organizations and graduate training programs. As we have seen, the industry urgently requires the health services research skills which faculty and graduate student involvement can provide. In turn, the training programs acquire adjunct clinical faculty to serve as preceptors, quality assured field training sites, and ongoing opportunities for field-based longitudinal research. Consumers are the beneficiaries of more precisely targeted interventions developed through outcome-oriented research. The day-to-day role of the network provider is extended formally to include role modeling, clinical supervision, student competency assessment, and health services research.

Finally, in this rapprochement, room will have to be found for two other significant players: the professional associations and the licensing and credentialing bodies. The advent and development of managed care—in all its variety—will ensure a wholesale restructuring of what it is to be a behavioral health care provider in a reformed system of health services organization and financing. Thus it is through the addition of these latter groups that governmental concerns about health professions and the public interest itself are formally addressed.

Without the associations' commitment to and active promulgation of practice standards and revised specialty accreditation criteria, accomplishment of the essentially utilitarian partnership of managed behavioral health care and the professional training programs will remain unformalized. It is the public interest that is, ostensibly, served by licensing and credentialing authorities. The codification of changes in the requisite armamentarium of behavioral health clinicians by such entities acts ultimately to consolidate the kind of changes in the nature of practice we have considered in this chapter.

What is of prime interest in this scenario is that the "arrow of change" with respect to professional roles and, consequently, of professional development is launched—not by professional associations, academic or licensing and credentialing bodies—but by the rapidly changing, chaotic, opportunistic and pragmatic industry of managed behavioral health care. It is past time for the entrenched players to catch up.

REFERENCES

Appelbaum, P.S. (1993). Legal liability and managed care. *American Psychologist, 48,* 251–257.

Austad, C.S., Sherman, W.O., Morgan, T., & Holstein, L. (1992). The psychotherapist and the managed care setting. *Professional Psychology: Research and Practice, 23,* 329–332.

Belar, C.D. (1989). Opportunities for psychologists in health maintenance organizations: Implications of graduate education and training. *Professional Psychology: Research and Practice, 20,* 390–394.

Belar, C.D. & Perry, N.W. (1992). National conference on scientist-practitioner education and training for the professional practice of psychology. *American Psychologist, 47,* 71–75.

Bent, R.J. (1986). Toward quality assurance in the education of practicing psychologists. In J.E. Callan, D.R. Peterson, & G. Stricker (Eds.), *Quality in Professional Psychology Training: A National Conference and Self-Study.* National Council of Schools of Professional Psychology, 27–36.

Blackwell, B. & Schmidt, G.L. (1992). Educational implications of managed mental health care. *Hospital and Community Psychiatry, 43,* 962–964.

Boaz, J.T. (1988). *Delivering Mental Healthcare: A Guide for HMOs.* Chicago: Pluribus Press.

Clements, C.B. (1992). Training in human service management for future practitioner-managers. *Professional Psychology: Research and Practice, 23,* 146–150.

Graham, S.R. & Fox, R.E. (1991). Postdoctoral education for professional practice. *American Psychologist, 46,* 1033–1035.

Hoshmand, L.T. & Polkinghorne, D.E. (1992). Redefining the science-practice relationship and professional training. *American Psychologist, 47,* 55–66.

Kiesler, C.A. (1992). U.S. mental health policy: Doomed to fail. *American Psychologist, 47,* 1077–1082.

Monahan, J. (1993). Limiting therapist exposure to Tarasoff liability: Guidelines for risk containment. *American Psychologist, 48,* 242–250.

Sharfstein, S.S. (1992). Managed mental health care. In A. Tasman & A.B. Riba

(Eds.), *Review of Psychiatry,* Volume 11. Washington, D.C.: American Psychiatric Press, Inc., 570–584.

VandenBos, G.R. (1993). U.S. mental health policy: Proactive evolution in the midst of health care reform. *American Psychologist, 48,* 289–290.

PART VI
SYSTEM ACCOUNTABILITY IN MANAGED CARE

PART VI: INTRODUCTORY NOTE

A likely eventuality is that, within the next decade, most health services will be provided by a relatively small number of very large managed care companies. This scenario suggests the critical role to be played by computer-based management information systems (MIS). As Rogerson explains in Chapter 11, a company can not grow beyond a modest size without access to an MIS. At the same time, the need for such a system extends beyond the case management process itself. It affects the company's capacity to properly manage its own activities, to monitor and assure the quality of the services it provides, and to be accountable to purchasers, consumers, and other stakeholders.

Because so many aspects of managed behavioral health care systems are complex, controversial, or developmental in their nature, the need for an organization to demonstrate accountability is paramount. Of particular interest currently is the issue of outcome or efficacy of the clinical services provided by the managed care company. As Pallak and Cummings state in Chapter 12, the capability of managed programs to collect and manipulate large sets of clinical data via a computer is a critical prerequisite to the development of a rigorous program of evaluation of clinical services. A second prerequisite is the availability of reliable and valid instruments which can be implemented, in a practical sense, in the everyday world of service delivery. In Pallak and Cummings' view, the technology exists, but what is needed is the willingness of managed care companies to make a commitment both to invest the resources necessary to support an adequate evaluation program and to be publicly accountable by publishing the data and allowing the audience to make judgments about the adequacy of the services provided by the organization.

The meta-issue, of course, relates to the adequacy of the managed care systems themselves to do what they proclaim they do better than traditional service delivery systems: save money as well as guarantee a certain level of quality. The public stance of these programs must be to generate the data necessary to demonstrate that they are doing the right thing and getting the right outcomes. It is frequently and compellingly argued, however, that definitive statements about the quality of these systems can only be made as a result of independent, external evaluation of their operation.

In Chapter 13 Milstein and his colleagues discuss their experiences as external evaluators examining the work of mental health and chemical dependency review organizations. The picture they paint is one of great variation and, from one perspective, unfulfilled promises of managed care. From another perspective, however, the chapter reflects an industry in relatively early developmental stages, characterized by experimentation and innovation, in which the "best practice models" are still to be determined.

Chapter 11

INFORMATION SYSTEM REQUIREMENTS FOR MANAGED CARE PROGRAMS

CHARLES L. ROGERSON

The feature of a managed behavioral health program perhaps most often associated with program quality by leaders in the industry is the automated management information system. Such systems can enable managed care programs to conduct effective and efficient case review and management while satisfying their clients' and sanctioners' needs for information about the quality and cost-effectiveness of the services provided by the system.

This chapter provides a rationale for automating a managed behavioral health program and delineates ways in which automation can support essential program activities. It also contains a discussion of the various functions of an automated system in the specific context of managed care, and provides guidelines for the development of such a system. Finally, it presents a description of an automated data system for a typical managed care program.

Why Automate Managed Mental Health Operations?

There are several major reasons for automating managed health care operations. They relate both to the internal efficiency of the operation and to the ability of the system to be responsive to the needs of its customers and sanctioners.

Reason 1: To Allow Growth

It is possible to operate a small managed behavioral health care program without an integrated information system. Three or four case managers can handle their case loads using paper case files, eligibility listings, "tickler" files, and provider network listings, but their effectiveness will be impaired by having to perform manual searches of these files and

193

lists. Even periodic reporting, on a small scale, can be done manually. Growth beyond a certain point, however, will be seriously impeded by the increase in volume and in time spent searching for files and extracting data for reports.

At some point, growth becomes impossible due to the flood of paper, the time spent searching for and through files, and the inability to report accurately on operations. Many managed care programs wait until they reach this point before managers begin seriously to deal with automation, by which time the pressure to do something can lead to injudicious decisions. The need to seek precipitous solutions may even lead the organization to delegate the decision-making authority to external consultants or to information system vendors. When considering automation, managed care program administrators should try to develop a good understanding of the current and future operational and reporting requirements of their system. This will increase the likelihood that the system eventually purchased will fit the business, rather than requiring the business to adapt to it.

Reason 2: To Increase Staff Effectiveness

A well-designed information system is capable of increasing the effectiveness and efficiency of case managers by providing them with improved access to information in a more useable (electronic rather than paper) form. More specifically, such a system can:

- substantially reduce the volume of paper files and lists which case managers must handle;
- reduce the time required to search for case files and eliminate instances of lost files;
- allow shared access to cases across case managers;
- reduce response time to queries from management, providers, and subscribers;
- improve communications among case managers;
- give case managers fast access to database tables of entities such as providers, facilities, diagnoses, and treatment plan summaries;
- automate access to criteria sets and assessment tools;
- automate the "tickler" or "next action date" function.

Reason 3: To Facilitate Management of the Program

A by-product of automation of the record-keeping and data-capture functions is access by program managers to a database describing in detail the operations of the program over time. This information can be reported and analyzed to improve, for example, managers' understanding of referral patterns, workloads, work flow, productivity, lag times, and bottlenecks. Improved oversight can result in more appropriate staffing and balancing of workloads, increased productivity, and the capacity to more accurately evaluate the cost of supporting specific client contracts.

Reason 4: To Improve Reporting Capabilities

Retaining existing clients and acquiring new clients are increasingly dependent on the capability of managed care programs to produce client reports which document savings, service quality, and outcomes. Such a capability requires a flexible reporting system that can generate both standard reports and special, *ad hoc,* reports to satisfy the unique needs of particular clients.

How Automation Supports Case Management Activities

Many case management activities are telephone-based. Since calls may be received from beneficiaries and providers at any time, on any case, reviewers must be able to use the information system to establish new cases, gain access to existing cases, and respond to queries—all in "real time." This requirement imposes many demands on the information system, demands which are exemplified in the following brief vignettes:

> *Example 1.* A provider returns a call from a reviewer on a case different from that which currently occupies the reviewer. The reviewer should be able to suspend the case he is working on, locate the one being referred to by the caller, resolve with the caller relevant issues, enter the relevant data into that record, and return to the original case—all with relative ease and speed.
> *Example 2.* In the course of consultation with a reviewer about a specific case, a provider asks about another of her cases which happens to be assigned to a second reviewer. The first reviewer should be able to access this other case, answer the provider's

question, make a notation about the contact or leave a message for the second reviewer, and then return to the original case without having to close and reopen the original case.

Example 3. While discussing a case with the utilization review (UR) nurse at a particular hospital, the case manager learns that the phone number of the hospital UR office has changed. The case manager needs to be able to access the record for the hospital, update the contact information, and return to the case being discussed with the UR nurse without losing her place in the case being discussed.

Example 4. A case manager who is speaking with a provider about treatment of a child also needs information about the treatment provided to the child's father. The case manager needs to be able to access the father's case without closing out the child's record.

In each of these four situations, it is crucial that the case manager in question has access as described, even if a second case manager is involved. Furthermore, as emphasized by use of statements such as "with relative ease", the details of the secondary case must be accessed with dispatch and with minimal effort on the part of the case manager. Systems which do not efficiently support a telephone-based work flow will be perceived by case managers as obstructive and will not be used. Rather, review personnel will continue to use paper forms requiring back-entering after phone calls are completed. If the volume of calls is large, data on the paper forms are likely to be forgotten, or lost, and never subsequently entered into the system. If a case manager does not have immediate and easy access to data necessary to answer a provider's question, redundant and irritating rounds of "phone tag" may ensue. Such inefficiencies significantly reduce productivity while undermining the integrity and completeness of the data needed to generate accurate and timely reports for management and clients.

The Functions of Automation

There are a number of specific requirements for functions which are unique to a managed care environment and which must be fulfilled by the automated system to render it maximally useful to the managed care program.

Providing Rapid, Shared Access to Multiple Databases

In their business relationships, managed programs deal with a large number of *entities* (Batini, Ceri, & Navathe, 1992). These entities may include clients (usually plan sponsors or payers), plans themselves, employers, employee groups, subscribers, members, providers, facilities, etc. The concept of entities is discussed in more detail below. At this point, it is important only to emphasize that since much of managed care involves brokering and managing relationships between and among these entities, it is crucial to have easily accessible and current information on them all, and to be able to link any of them with specific cases.

Within the information system, data about entities should be organized into tables by entity type (plan, provider, etc.), with records in each table containing summary and detailed information on each specific individual entity. For example, there should be a *client table* with a record for each (corporate) client, and a *provider table* with a record for each psychiatrist, psychologist, social worker, and any other type of individual provider. These tables should be easily accessible at any time during the processing of a case. They should also be simple to update, so that when, for example, a social worker calls with a new telephone number for his office, this record can immediately and easily be changed.

Establishing, Tracking, and Maintaining Cases

The fundamental entity in any program which performs review or case management is the *case* —a record of services delivered to a subscriber by any network provider or facility and actions, such as referrals, taken by staff. Reviewers must be able to use the automated system to initiate a case quickly and easily while they are engaged in a telephone conversation with a provider or subscriber. They must be able to verify or capture necessary data items, enter notes, and set up "next action" or "tickler" dates. When a call is received on an open (already existing) case, it should be simple for the person answering the call to locate that case, ascertain the reviewer responsible for the case, and transfer the call to the appropriate reviewer. If the reviewer is unavailable, the person taking the call should be able to access the case, answer a query, and update the record or make a note, as required.

Since cases are necessarily dynamic, and since complex cases may involve multiple professional providers or facilities at different times, the information system should support case journals in which updates to the case are recorded and time-, date-, and user-stamped. This type of journaling allows rapid reconstruction of the course of a case, a record which would otherwise have to be laboriously extracted from the case notes.

Supporting the Case Management Process

As much as possible, the information system should be compatible with the full range of operational activities of the particular managed care program it is designed to serve. Not only must it allow easy access to critical information concerning the entities with which the company has business connections, it also must support a variety of business functions and operations, particularly the case management function.

For example, if the company performs telephone referrals to providers for subscribers who inquire about mental health or substance abuse services, the system should permit immediate verification of subscriber eligibility. It should also facilitate the triage function: the development of a diagnosis and estimation of problem severity (possibly by use of an automated decision-making process), and identification of an appropriate level of care (LOC). It should allow also the identification of a provider for the designated LOC (e.g., acute care facility, outpatient practitioner) in the subscriber's service area and, under some circumstances, may be used to schedule appointments. If the case management process involves the evaluation of treatment plans, the system should support such assessments and be capable of capturing the results of these evaluations for subsequent aggregation and reporting.

Supporting the Use and Development of Criteria

Processes of triage, LOC evaluation, referral, and treatment plan evaluation involve the use of either implicit or explicit criteria. Although such evaluations will always involve professional judgment, the use of explicit, written criteria improves the consistency (i.e., reliability) of review decisions. The consistency provided by explicit criteria is important not only when dealing with individual providers with routine case matters, but also in exceptional situations such as when a review or case management decision is appealed.

In medical/surgical review and case management, there are several explicit criteria sets in wide use (Gertman & Restuccia, 1982; Doyle, 1992; InterQual, 1992). Criteria sets for behavioral health programs have only recently been developed, and are significantly less comprehensive.

Nonetheless, an automated information system in behavioral health should be able to support those criteria which are in place and permit the addition and modification of criteria as they are developed and implemented.

Criteria relevant to a case should be available to reviewers both for phone conversations with providers or subscribers, and while they are reviewing documents such as treatment plans or case reports which have been submitted by providers. If the criteria are embedded in a "flowchart" or decision tree, the logical process of decision-making should be supported by the automated system.

Supporting Provider Network Administration

A key component of a managed care program is the provider network. This system usually has two components: an organized group of independently practicing professionals, which may include marriage and family counselors, clinical social workers, psychiatric nurses, psychologists, and psychiatrists; and a group of facilities and programs such as psychiatric hospitals, psychiatric wards of general acute care hospitals, inpatient detoxification units, residential and outpatient drug rehabilitation programs, and residential treatment centers for children and adolescents. The provider and facility networks should cover the full spectrum of types and levels of care and should provide good geographic coverage. Developing, maintaining, and evaluating these networks is a complex and challenging process that is virtually impossible without automation.

The automated system should support network administration by centralizing provider information in professional and facility tables which contain data required by both case managers and provider relations personnel. Network administration should be integrated with the review and management functions of the managed care program.

Case managers, who are in daily contact with providers and facilities, require up-to-date information on the network and are usually the first persons in the system to become aware of changes in phone numbers or addresses. Case management staff, therefore, should have ready access to information about the network and should be able to directly enter changes and notes about the providers into the system.

Supporting Provider Profiling

Increasingly, developers of managed care programs are coming to realize the crucial importance of evaluating the performance of providers in their networks. In the early days of managed care, networks were developed simply to ensure discounted fees and geographic coverage. Even credentialing received little attention, and the attention that it was accorded was due primarily to concerns about legal liability.

More recently, managed care programs and their clients have been demonstrating increasing concern about the quality of care delivered by network providers. It has become clear to all such organizations that, despite their complexity, quality assurance issues must be given appropriate emphasis. These factors are even playing a significant role in the marketing of managed care programs.

Every managed care program should have serious, continuous quality assessment and improvement functions. The information system should support these functions by facilitating the development of reports concerning diagnoses or other forms of problem definition, service components, quality incidents, and provider profiles. The use of such reports allows the program to monitor and assess the patterns and quality of care provided by individual providers and programs for specific problems or conditions.

Supporting Flexible Report Generation

Generally, reporting is seen as an output of the system, as a by-product of operations. Because of this, it is often the last function to be considered in system design (as it is in this chapter). Despite this authorial lapse, it is the development of reporting requirements for the managed care program which should be the initial consideration in order to ensure that both the data elements and the data structures essential to report generation are included in the system design from the outset.

A common problem for managed care programs is that reporting requirements are less well understood than are the operational requirements, primarily because the demand for reports generally evolves over time. Consequently, report specifications are commonly not available to system designers. In addition, reporting needs in managed care are continually expanding in response to research/evaluation needs and market demands. It is also true that clients demand increasingly sophisticated reports and are less and less willing to accept statements about operational savings, quality, and effectiveness without empirical evidence for these claims. Therefore, the information system must be able to produce not only standard reports, but also *ad hoc* reports and data extracts for statistical analysis.

Structure of the Entity Database

After committing to the decision to automate the managed care program or to upgrade or replace an existing information system, program managers should perform the exercise of listing and defining all entities with which the program is involved in the course of doing business. These entities will include, but are not limited to, clients, employer groups, plans, subscribers, members, providers, contracts, and treatment plans. These entities have attributes (e.g., name, unique identification number, address, eligibility status, specialty) which need to be recognized by the program in the course of operations. Attributes should be listed and defined for each entity. The different relationships that exist between and among these entities should also be listed. For example, professional providers deliver a variety of particular professional services to members; case reviewers process member requests for services; and the program reports on its activities to clients.

Clearly, the process of entity analysis could continue almost indefinitely. How far does it need to go? It should be kept in mind that the primary goal is the development of an information system that supports the complexities of case management. The analysis should, therefore, continue until:

- all entities with which the managed care program comes in contact in the course of doing business have been defined;
- their attributes have been defined to the level of detail required by business operations; and
- their relationships to each other have been defined to an extent that reflects their business relationships and the program's business operations.

This analysis should be done as the first step in developing a request for proposal—a document which will become the basis for recruiting the vendor or company which will supply or develop the information system.

In evaluating system solutions proposed by vendors, or when designing an in-house system, attention should be given to the extent to which the system deals with each entity, whether it captures the necessary attributes of each entity, and whether the system functions match the relationships between the entities and the operations of the managed care program. The definitive question should be how well the automated system actually mirrors the managed care program in structure, content, and process. It is not necessary for the system to capture data on every entity and support every relationship. The managed service system, for example, is probably not applicable to the automation of office supplies inventories. It is clearly preferable, however, to perform an exhaustive analysis, and then discard certain entities or functions, than to have to contend with the consequences of an incomplete initial analysis.

One systems approach which has been employed successfully in the past is to use a *relational database* tool to create a file, or table in relational terms, for each entity. Together these tables make up the entity database. For example, there would be a client table and a facility table. Each table would contain one record, or row, for each individual client or facility. Each row would consist of the data elements, or attributes, common to all instances of that entity. For subscribers, these attributes would include data such as name, social security number, address, phone, and date of birth. Figure 1 contains a list of entities and their attributes that are typically involved in a managed care program.

Conclusion

Without the capabilities provided by automated management information systems, the capacity of managed mental health programs to grow, to function competitively, to ensure quality, and to be accountable to their customers and sanctioners is significantly diminished. There is no doubt that the promise of managed care will not be realized without the availability of comprehensive and flexible automated systems which effectively serve both the internal (case management) and external (accountability) purposes of these programs.

An automated system, regardless of its scope, appropriateness, flexibility, and operational parsimony, can not guarantee the quality of managed care. The absence of such a system, however, will guarantee the failure of the program to achieve the level of quality demanded by increasingly sophisticated purchasers of managed care and others who sanction provider services on behalf of their clients.

Figure 1

Entities and Associated Attributes in a Managed Care Program

ENTITY	ATTRIBUTES

CASE	Case manager ID
	User-assigned reference ID
	Type
	Category code (out of area, mental health, CD, etc.)
	Status code
	Pointers to:
	      member
	      provider(s)
	      facility (ies)
	      diagnoses
	      procedures
	      group
	      plan
	Date opened, type/reason code
	Date of onset/injury
	Date of first provider contact, type of contact code
	Date of last contact, type of contact code
	Most recent action
	Level of Care
	Visits: requested, approved, used
	LOS: requested, approved, used
	Next action date (tickler)
	Case notes

SUBSCRIBER	Reference ID Type Demographics Notes
MEMBER	As for subscriber
CLIENT COMPANY	Reference ID Type Identifying and contact data Notes
CARRIER	As for client company
EMPLOYER	As for carrier (above)
EMPLOYEE GROUP	As for carrier (above)
PLAN	As for carrier (above) Plan summary
FACILITY/PROGRAM	Reference ID Type Identifying data Contact data Notes
SERVICE PROVIDER	As for facility Specialty
DIAGNOSIS	Type Category Code Descriptor
PROCEDURE	As for diagnosis

REFERENCES

Batini, C., Ceri, S., & Navathe, S.B. (1992). *Conceptual Database Design: An Entity-Relationship Approach.* Redwood City, CA: Benjamin-Cummings Publishing.

Doyle, R. (1992). *Healthcare Management Guidelines.* Seattle: Milliman & Robertson.

InterQual (1992). *The ISD-A™ Review System with ISD-A™ Criteria.* North Hampton, NH: InterQual.

Gertman, P.M., & Restuccia, J.D. (1981). Appropriateness Evaluation Protocol: A technique for assessing unnecessary days of hospital care. *Medical Care, 19,* 855–871.

Chapter 12

OUTCOMES RESEARCH IN MANAGED BEHAVIORAL HEALTH CARE: ISSUES, STRATEGIES, AND TRENDS

Michael S. Pallak and Nicholas A. Cummings

At least three factors fuel the current wave of enthusiasm for research on clinical outcome and clinical effectiveness in the behavioral health care industry. By far the most important factor is the continuing rise in costs for alcohol, drug abuse, and mental health services—the same cost trends which gave the initial impetus to managed care. A second factor is the perception within the managed care industry that evidence about outcome treatment effectiveness may be useful for marketing purposes in the competition for services contracts. The third factor relates to the increasing availability of useful and practical measurement instruments and strategies which may be adapted to behavioral health services research in managed care settings.

In this chapter, we explore the implications of these factors for clinical outcome research and examine strategies and tools needed to conduct such efforts. Each of the three factors may represent either an impetus or a barrier to empirical evaluation of clinical outcome, depending upon how organizations judge the relative values of the cost of conducting research and the utility of the outcome results for marketing and operating purposes. Each factor may also motivate or enable patients, insurers, and employers to ask more astute questions about whether services provided are in fact clinically effective as well as financially viable. The growing emphasis on outcome and effectiveness data represents a major shift in perspective on the part of buyers of managed behavioral health care services.

205

INDUSTRY TRENDS: EVOLUTION IN RESPONSE TO COST

Unfortunately, mental health services and related policy have been secondary concerns and poor relations to medical-surgical services and policy for most of this century. The shape of health services delivery and policies affecting their development and implementation has primarily been driven by funding issues related to medical-surgical hospitals rather than by the more comprehensive range of issues which should appropriately affect national health policy and priorities (Klerman, 1985; Stevens, 1989; Kiesler, 1991). Based on Stevens (1989), Kiesler (1991) argues that the fact that 70% of each mental health treatment dollar is spent on inpatient services is a result of a long history of policy in which hospitalization is—inappropriately—construed as the primary treatment modality in health as well as mental health.

Cost as a Factor

Costs in both medical and behavioral health care have continued to increase at a rate faster than inflation, population increase, or growth in GNP would predict. In the 1970s and 1980s, cost increases prompted the development by payers of a range of cost containment strategies, most of which were implemented as benefit restrictions and other barriers to care. These strategies failed to control costs of mental health and chemical dependency on a long-term basis (Cummings, 1991).

The failure of the cost containment strategies led to attempts by payers and service organizations to redefine service delivery models, combining clinical provision of services with a business-oriented management of those services. The business "bottom-line" orientation provided impetus for an outcome perspective in terms of financial profit. The simultaneous desire to "manage" the service delivery led organizations to attempt to address the broader cost-effectiveness question: *Can clinically effective treatment be delivered at lower levels of intensity and, therefore, lower cost?*

With this change in perspective came a questioning of the previously unquestioned assumption that usual patterns of treatment were automatically necessary and automatically clinically effective. A more evaluative or outcome-focused orientation came to predominate. The potential for rising costs to erode profitability brought into question, for example, whether the observed clinical outcomes justified the relatively high utilization levels of inpatient treatment.

While the managers were beginning to ask cost-effectiveness questions, researchers were contributing to the shifting perspective by presenting a growing body of empirical research which showed that less costly and less intensive levels of care were generally equally effective in terms of patient outcomes. Kiesler & Sibulkin (1987), for example, reviewed a large number of experimental studies in which mental health patients were randomly assigned either to inpatient treatment or to any one of several outpatient treatment alternatives. Patients assigned to the alternative outpatient treatment did as well as those assigned to the more routinely prescribed inpatient care, almost always at less cost.

In another review, Kiesler & Morton (1988) found that length of stay in an inpatient psychiatric facility was more accurately predicted by variables unrelated (exogenous) to the patient's condition than by endogenous variables such as severity of illness. Kerns & Bradley (1990) provided an extensive and detailed analysis of clinician, patient, and system factors which had been shown to have an impact on the decision to hospitalize. Finally, research on outpatient treatment cast doubt on the cost-effectiveness of anything more than about 24 sessions for the typical psychotherapy or counseling patient (Howard, Kopta, Krause, & Orlinsky, 1986). In short, the growing body of research literature questioned the cost-effectiveness of the more intensive and longer-term services for all but a small percentage of the patients who typically received them.

As sophistication about outcome and efficacy issues increased among payers and service organizations, a primary service objective was reconceptualized as one of matching the patient to the intensity and level of care most appropriate for his or her condition. This was a much more proactive stance than had been typical of these organizations. For example, in one case study, Pallak & Cummings (1992) found that 85% of patients presenting for inpatient admission could be successfully redirected to intensive outpatient treatment.

In this environment, as costs continued to rise and as competition in the marketplace increased, payers and purchasers of health and mental health services became better able and increasingly motivated to routinely ask the outcome questions: *Are the services provided clinically effective?* and *Are there equally effective but less costly alternatives for the patient?* The relatively straightforward goal of reducing or restraining the rate of increase in costs, typically by restricting access to services, gave way to the much more complex task of ensuring that purchased services were cost-effective. Purchasers of mental health services increasingly attempted to base their contracting decisions on consideration of clinical effectiveness as well as cost.

Competition as a Factor

Competition among providers of systems of care is increasingly important as a factor in the managed care industry's move toward providing evidence for the clinical effectiveness of their services. In essence, the question is no longer merely whether a provider organization can mount a program of service delivery for a specific number of covered lives, but also whether the organization will be able to document the clinical effectiveness of those services to the satisfaction of the purchaser. In very simple terms, service organizations must be able to demonstrate in a way that makes sense to the third party payer or (increasingly) the employer that the services make a positive difference in the patient's functional status.

Challenges in Addressing Outcome Issues

Managed care companies face three problems when attempting to develop and implement processes to address treatment effectiveness: (1) inertia and orientation of the managed care organization; (2) difficulty in defining outcomes; and (3) difficulty measuring outcome in typical clinical settings in an efficient and easily implemented fashion.

Inertia and Orientation of Managed Care Organization

Certain characteristics shared by most managed care organizations tend to reduce the likelihood that these companies will be either motivated to address outcome issues or capable of doing so.

INERTIA DUE TO FINANCIAL ORIENTATION. To the extent that a strict business, accounting, or insurance perspective dominates the managed care organization, an outcome orientation and questions of treatment effectiveness will probably remain relatively distant concerns. The typical industry standard for information in an insurance or other third party program is fairly simple claims data. Such data are most useful on an actuarial basis for ascertaining how much and what types of treatments were authorized, delivered, and paid for. In this context, the industry simply tracks services which are paid for and leaves judgments about effectiveness and outcome of treatment to the individual provider, the patient, or others. This straightforward approach is primarily geared to financial management to determine, for example, what needs to be charged for the product in the next financial cycle in order to maintain profitability.

A claims data system can, however, be a fundamental element in the process of monitoring and evaluating the service system. Depending on level of detail captured in the data base, claims data can be used to assess factors that shape service utilization and patterns of service delivery. For example, the observed striking variations in patterns of inpatient utilization within the same clinical diagnosis (Kiesler & Morton, 1988) suggest that factors other than the patient's condition drive inpatient service utilization. While even these simple sorts of analyses can be useful in evaluating the services system, they are not likely to be conducted when the information system and staff are oriented solely to claims paid and financial goals.

INERTIA DUE TO A "SIMPLE" QA ORIENTATION. A variety of process-focused review and quality assurance (QA) procedures have evolved within the health services industry. QA procedures and criteria-based review combined with an adequate information system allow tracking of services delivered and assessment of whether "appropriate" (as defined by criteria) care was delivered at appropriate points in time. When combined with information from outcome assessment, such systems provide both a critical monitoring function and a tool by which the process as well as the structure of service provision may be shaped. For example, the review process maintained within an outcome-focused quality assurance program allows the determination of conditions under which morbidity or mortality are more likely to be observed and provides the organization with an empirical basis for making changes in the structure or process of treatment to reduce risk and the probability of adverse consequences.

As typically implemented, however, the QA process represents a partial, but largely inadequate, evaluation of treatment outcome and effectiveness. Under such a process, patterns of treatment are examined, criteria and standards or norms for treatment provision are developed, causes for deviations are analyzed, and changes are implemented to minimize probability of deviations in the future. This "simple" QA system permits aggregation of relevant information across providers, patients, and services settings as a basis for evaluating primarily the *process* of service delivery.

The inherent problem with this type of QA, of course, is that procedural refinements in the process of service delivery do not necessarily translate into better treatment outcomes. This can only happen if appropriate measures of treatment outcome are added to the information routinely collected as part of QA so that the "process-outcome links" can be established. In the most stereotyped example, all the correct steps in the process of treatment provision may have unfolded (according to the criteria), but the average patient may not have improved or been fully restored to functioning. The critical unanswered question is, *What aspects of the process were responsible for the treatment failure?* The situation is particularly problematic in systems where the evidence from the empirical assessment of patient outcome is not routinely available to the QA program, existing, at best, in the unexamined and unquantified case notes contained in the patient's chart and, at worst, only in the mind of the individual service providers.

INERTIA DUE TO A SIMPLE "SELLING" ORIENTATION. For service delivery organizations, marketplace issues and the need to be competitive may conflict with the need or desire to evaluate treatment effectiveness. On the one hand, a simple "selling" orientation requires making the best, if not superlative, case for the provider organization and what it offers in terms of services. From this perspective, considerations of treatment effectiveness, which necessarily include analysis of "failures" and variations in outcomes, may not represent the strongest selling position and, as a result, may not be viewed as a priority for allocation of in-house resources.

In contrast, an organization with an outcome orientation focuses on instances of both positive and less than positive outcome as a means to understand the treatment process and the outcome-process relationships and to develop more effective clinical procedures. Sophisticated efforts are often necessary to evaluate treatment and clinical outcomes, and organizations which commit to such an approach also must be willing to commit sufficient resources to support the activities.

Both selling and outcomes perspectives can be accommodated if the buyer as well as the managed care company take a more analytical approach to the utilization of outcome data. For example, the fact that chemical dependency and substance abuse services are less than 100% effective may lead to a more enlightened discussion about the relative value and necessity of more complex treatment procedures in order to maximize the percentage of patients who remain abstinent at treatment follow-up. Such a discussion could result in more realistic expectations about outcome on the part of the buyer, and to a cooperative effort between buyer and seller to obtain or develop alternative models of service or support for particular types of patients.

Despite the inertias, the simple computerized data system and QA program maintained by most managed care companies provide a reasonable basis from which to develop approaches to the issues of treatment outcome and treatment effectiveness in systems of care. At the same time, marketplace trends and competitive pressures in the industry will force increased attention to the more complex issues of patient outcomes. This will be the major focus of development in QA within existing service delivery systems for the next three to five years. The impetus will be the need to answer both the "simple" QA question (*Was the treatment appropriately delivered?*) and the more "complex" questions (*What was the treatment outcome?* and *What aspects of treatment process were related to the outcome?*).

Measuring Treatment Outcome

Given the rather poor record of managed behavioral health care systems in evaluating outcomes, one would be forgiven for believing that the techniques and procedures for doing so have not kept pace with the rapid evolution of the managed systems themselves. In fact, measures and technologies have existed for some time, but only recently have they been adopted or applied, as the importance of quantifying and evaluating treatment outcome has come to be realized within the managed care industry (Pallak, 1989). Still, however, the empirical research base for behavioral health services (as for behavioral sciences more generally) has largely remained outside of the business environment, within research and academic settings (Pallak & Kilburg, 1986; Pallak, 1989).

There are a number of factors that have contributed to the absence of research applications to the world of service delivery and policy development in general (Kaschau, Rehm & Ullman, 1985). In addition, there have been several sources of inertia reinforcing the historical separation between the research "industry" concerned with behavioral health services and the behavioral health service delivery systems themselves.

A major source probably lies with the stereotypes emanating from the psychoanalytic roots of mental health treatment. According to this admittedly simplified view, clinical services of necessity involve intensive treatment (three to five times per week) over several years with the objective of "deep" or "fundamental" personality change, rarely quantifiable (and not easily documented, in any event). In light of these implicit definitions of outcome, any change in personality *function* (that is, changes which could be measured), as opposed to *structure,* in response to treatment was often viewed as evidence of superficial rather than "real change" and not worth measuring in any systematic fashion. For a myriad of reasons, many of these related to the exigencies of health care financing, the psychoanalytic view has lost influence within the mental health community. It has been displaced by new approaches, exemplified by the theories of Aaron Beck (Beck, Hollon, Young et al., 1985). These new approaches are more structured and directive than psychoanalytic methods, and they are, therefore, much more suited to outcome investigations focused on objective and measurable changes.

Two factors facilitated the movement toward investigations of clinical treatment outcome in applied settings. The first was the growing body of evidence that mental health treatment actually "works". This is best exemplified by the Smith, Glass, and Miller (1980) meta-analytic approach to analyzing therapy outcomes. This research strategy indicated that across a variety of studies, in a variety of settings, using a variety of treatment approaches and measures, patients treated with psychotherapy show improvement relative to controls.

The second factor is the increasing sophistication of psychotherapy research in terms of measures and techniques used to assess outcomes. While some clinical or psychotherapy research studies (Battle et al., 1966) rely on relatively simple measures targeted to the initial problem (indeed, this was the dominant model for many years), more recent studies, typified by the work of Luborsky and his colleagues, involve intensive procedures for data collection and analysis focused on both the process and the outcome of treatment (Luborsky et al., 1988). Combinations of patient questionnaires, provider ratings of clinical progress, ratings by third party clinical judges, and periodic structured interviews have been used to study in depth the process-outcome links. Their results demonstrate that patients improve with treatment, but they also suggest that combinations of patient and provider factors are likely to facilitate or retard clinical improvement. Through efforts of researchers such as Luborsky, the more general debate about whether psychotherapy "works", has been replaced by an evaluative focus on the conditions under which psychotherapy and mental health treatment may be effective (i.e., what combinations of treatment approaches, treatment providers or settings, patients, and problems lead to improvement, and how that improvement can be documented).

The Patient's Perceptions

A patient's perception of his or her progress in coping with problems and restoration of function is a critical measure of clinical effectiveness. For example, Battle et al. (1966) argued that patients seek help with problems and "target" complaints and therefore, just as in medical settings, treatment effectiveness should be judged by whether the patient believes the problem has been alleviated. In their procedure, Battle et al. (1966) asked patients to write in their own words the three problems they most wanted help with and how severe these problems were. At completion of the treatment episode patients were asked again to rate the problems in terms of severity. Change in the patient's rating of the severity was shown to be a useful indicator of patient improvement and clinical effectiveness.

Patient reactions, judgments, and perceptions of their status and well-being have long been recognized by clinicians themselves as important (perhaps the most important) indicators of clinical effectiveness. For example, in a meeting with some 300 clinical providers of all types during 1991, the clinicians were asked how they knew that their patients improved. The unanimous response was that the patients report improvement directly, in their own words, about developing better coping strategies and about handling problems differently.

A patient's satisfaction with treatment and perception of treatment effectiveness in terms of his or her ability to more effectively deal with problems are critical indicators for a service system. Patients who perceive little progress or report low levels of satisfaction with the services are patients whom we want to know about, since they are the ones most likely to provide the system with information useful in quality improvement efforts.

While there are a variety of general and specific measures of patient outcome, this chapter is not intended as a detailed review or handbook. Rather, the interested reader is referred to resources such as the Health and Psychosocial Instrument (HAPI) data base file (Perloff, 1991) which includes detailed information (reliability, validity, availability, etc.) about a range of specific instruments.

There are a number of short, general measures such as the Client Satisfaction Questionnaire (Nguyen, Attkisson, & Stegner, 1983) which have excellent validity and correlate well with patients' decision to complete treatment. These more general instruments are particularly useful in applied clinical settings, since they may be easily administered in 5–10 minutes (for example, after any treatment session), or can be mailed as follow-up questionnaires after the treatment episode is completed. Periodic administration of brief measures has the advantage of permitting a view of the treatment process over time that may be easily correlated with particular events of clinical interest.

Most questionnaires can be adapted for optically scanned scoring so their results can be directly entered into a data base. This allows the data to be easily summarized and otherwise manipulated as part of, for example, a QA program, and correlated or matched with treatment and other patient information. Organizations such as National Computer Services, Inc. can provide most instruments in optically scannable form along with normative information for the instrument. (See the list of resources at the end of this chapter.) For any particular patient or subgroup of patients, one can quickly establish clinical functioning in relation to other patient or norm groups, and can track change in functioning either on an "own control" basis (how the patient scores relative to his or her rating at earlier points in time) or relative to other patients with specific characteristics of interest. These scores can be aggregated for the entire service system or for particular components (e.g., for particular provider groups or programs) as one indication of how the service delivery system functions in whole or in part.

Treatment Outcome Measures: New Trends

In recent years there have been two trends of significance in the development of instruments and their application as outcome measures. The first is the use of general "health status" measures to evaluate outcome of behavioral health, as well as other health, treatment. These instruments are exemplified by the Health Status Questionnaire (HSQ) developed initially for the RAND Health Insurance Experiment (Ware, 1991; Brook, Ware, Davies-Avery et al., 1979). The second trend has been a growing emphasis on evaluating patient functioning and well-being (Ellwood, 1988) by focusing on configurations of problems and patterns of behavior specific to various diagnoses. These two trends have been facilitated by the work of Ellwood's InterStudy group who have given impetus to a variety of useful measures and strategies in applied health care settings.

THE HEALTH STATUS QUESTIONNAIRE. The Health Status Questionnaire (Ware & Sherbourne, 1991) consists of 36 items that represent eight dimensions of patient functioning: physical functioning, social functioning, role limitations due to physical problems, role limitations due to emotional problems, general mental health status, vitality, bodily pain, and general perceptions of own health. It is based on the assumption that a person's sense of well-being is impaired by emotional distress and that improvement in well-being is a useful outcome measure in the treatment of mental and emotional problems. The HSQ has excellent validity and involves only a minimum of patient time to complete (about 10–15 minutes). It is sufficiently sensitive to detect changes in patient responses, either in terms of a global factor (well-being) or on more specific dimensions. A score or scores on this measure can be easily added to existing QA data, thereby "closing the loop" in terms of patient outcomes that are easily quantified.

ASSESSING PATTERNS OF BEHAVIOR. Equally exciting are the activities of the InterStudy organization (Ellwood, 1988) which has supported the development of instruments focused on the assessment of configurations of problems and patterns of behavior more specific to various diagnoses (e.g., alcohol abuse, depression). These TyPE (Technology of Patient Experience) measures have demonstrated substantial potential for measuring outcomes and change due to treatment in most clinical settings. As such, they show promise of becoming a standard industry gauge. InterStudy supports an extensive program of instrument development and refinement and encourages data sharing among organizations using its instruments. The TyPE measures may be used alone or with other measures tailored to particular treatment settings, thereby providing a comprehensive profile of outcomes in terms of national as well as local or specific trends.

EMERGENCE OF EXTERNAL EVALUATORS. Another important development in research in managed care has been the rise of independent groups or firms able to conduct outcome evaluations on a contract basis for organizations which provide services. There are several compelling reasons for the existence of such firms, not the least of which is that managed care companies are often reluctant to devote financial resources to support internal evaluation efforts. Many companies regard research and evaluation activities as inconsistent with their business and marketing-oriented mission. As a result, overhead costs associated with the collection, processing, and interpretation of clinical data are seen as prohibitive to undertaking these activities.

A second reason relates to the lack of rigor with which internal outcome evaluations are often conducted. Much of the outcome data generated internally may be in the form of cases studies, may be descriptive, or may be correlational in nature. If they are not experimental, studies may not be considered rigorous enough to be meaningful. For example, they often would not be acceptable to peer reviewed academic journals. At best, they may require replications which involve additional costs to the managed care company.

Perhaps, more importantly, the data generated internally are considered proprietary and often, of course, reflect at least some outcomes which are less than perfect. Managed care companies (and especially their marketing departments) may well be reluctant to publish data indicating that the services may need improvement.

A final reason for development of external evaluations, and the one which is probably most commonly used publicly as justification for not conducting evaluations internally, is the belief that the objectivity of the results of internal efforts would be questioned—that is, positive results would be seen as self-serving if produced from the managed care company's own internal operations. This is always an issue in the marketplace ruled by fierce competition for service-delivery contracts, and it exemplifies the sharp divergence between the world of business and that of research. In the research world, work is driven by a search for truth. Publication in independently peer-reviewed outlets provides checks and balances on the rigor, quality, and replicability of research studies. In the business world, considerations over and above the search for truth drive decisions about internally supported evaluation—whether to do it, what to do, and whether and where to publish it.

As a consequence of this situation, firms such as Strategic Advantage Inc. (Naditch, 1989) have been organized to provide outcome evaluations on a contract basis. With this type of approach, the client organization need not build the internal capacity to mount its own research or evaluation efforts. While it is argued that these types of externally conducted efforts are more likely to be objective and less likely to be seen as self-serving, there is still some potential for bias if, for example, the outside evaluator wishes to develop a long-term relationship with the client organization.

Considering Medical Offset

Researchers focusing on outcome research in behavioral health services have moved toward a broader definition of outcome. In particular, much attention has been given to investigating the changes in the patient's utilization of medical services which may be related to the need for substance abuse or mental health services (Cummings & Follette, 1968; Jones & Vischi, 1979; Schlesinger, Mumford, Glass et al., 1983; Pallak, 1989). In general, it has been shown that many patients who seek behavioral health treatment exhibit patterns of increasing medical services utilization leading up to the time of receiving mental health or substance abuse treatment. The use of medical services typically lessens following treatment for the behavioral health problems.

The usual explanation for the "offset" effect is that emotional distress (and, sometimes, associated substance abuse) may exacerbate physical and medical conditions, or may lead to increased somaticization of the distress, thereby leading to increased utilization of medical services. According to this theory, treatment of the distress will result in a decline in medical services utilization and the cost of such services. Therefore, a reduction in medical services utilization following behavioral health treatment may be taken as an indicator of effect of that treatment. This may be particularly true for patients who are high medical utilizers, who have chronic medical conditions, or who have medical conditions exacerbated by high levels of emotional distress. Furthermore, assertively channelling high medical utilizers into behavioral health treatment may represent an area of longer term cost savings particularly for patients with chronic medical diagnoses (Pallak, 1989; Pallak, Cummings, Dörken & Henke, 1991).

There are some difficulties involved in attempting to use medical services utilization data, such as physician office visits, hospital days, and drug prescriptions, as an index of clinical effectiveness of behavioral health services. A major one is that mental health and substance abuse claim files must be merged with medical services claim files, if, as is often true, they are separate or are managed by different groups under the insurance plan, and utilization must be tracked over time. Second, an effect may not be apparent if data are aggregated into, for example, a single calendar year summary. Rather, medical services utilization needs to be tracked in appropriate units of time before and after the initiation of the behavioral health treatment. The advantage of using medical services utilization data lies in the fact that the data collection process is non-intrusive for the patient, and the data constitute an objective and empirical measure of outcome.

Treatment Outcomes Research: Some Observations

Current measures and technologies make it feasible to assess on a routine basis the outcomes of treatment provided in a wide variety of clinical settings. General measures of the patient's perceptions of treatment outcome as well as measures specific to particular clinical conditions are available, easily implemented, and easily incorporated into computerized data bases and QA systems before, during, and after treatment episodes. Many of these measures are excellent from a psychometric perspective, and they frequently are associated with normative data that can be useful for making judgments about profiles of patients, providers, treatment settings, and other variables of interest. Adding these types of data routinely to QA programs allows the service system to establish a relatively sophisticated picture of the relationship between the clinical process and patient outcomes.

Whether managed care companies exploit the potential of these available tools on a routine basis will be determined by the interaction among several factors. While the development of an outcome approach is feasible given the available technology, system inertias and the resources required to make a commitment to outcomes research act as mitigating factors.

The likely compromise for many managed care companies will be to mount small outcome evaluation efforts conducted by external organizations specializing in applied research and evaluation. Since much of the motivation for conducting outcomes analysis stems from marketplace pressure and business competition, many managed care providers will probably be content with limited short-term projects to demonstrate a commitment to accountability. These studies will be largely conducted for marketing purposes—to enable a provider to claim successful clinical outcomes relative to competitors. Eventually each provider group will probably have a "showcase" study, and potential buyers will be left once again to judge the quality of the results presented and to gauge the implications of the results for their specific beneficiary population or group.

The ultimate gauge of quality of results and, consequently, the value of those results for judging the quality of the services, will be whether or not these studies appear in peer reviewed publication outlets rather than only in marketing presentations. The most likely best outcome for the industry will be represented by managed care companies that invest in a modest but serious routine internal research and evaluation capacity for collection of outcome data, and supplement this with periodic intensive evaluations of those data conducted on a project basis by research and evaluation specialists.

REFERENCES

Battle, C., Imber, S.D., Hoehn-Saric, L.A., Stone, A.R., Nash, E.H., & Frank, J.D. (1966). Target complaints as criteria of improvement. *American Journal of Psychotherapy, 20,* 184–92.

Beck, A.T., Hollon, S.D., Young, J.E. et al. (1985). Treatment of depression with cognitive therapy and amitriptyline. *Archives of General Psychiatry, 42,* 142–148.

Brook, R.H., Ware, J.E., Davies-Avery, A. et al. (1979). Overview of adult health status measures fielded in RAND's health insurance study. *Medical Care, 19,* 787.

Cummings, N.A. (1991). Ten ways to spot mismanaged mental health care. *Psychotherapy in Private Practice, 9,* 31–33.

Cummings, N.A. & Follette, W.T. (1968). Psychiatric services and medical utilization in a prepaid health plan setting: Part II. *Medical Care, 6,* 31–41.

Ellwood, P.M. (1988). Outcomes management: A technology of patient experience. *New England Journal of Medicine, 318,* 1549.

Howard, K., Kopta, S., Krause, M., & Orlinsky, D. (1986). The dose-effect relationship in psychotherapy. *American Psychologist, 41,* 159–164.

Jones, K. & Vischi, T. (1979). The impact of alcohol, drug abuse and mental health treatment on medical care utilization: A review of the research literature. *Medical Care, 17,* #12, Supplement.

Kasschau, R.A., Rehm, L.P., & Ullman, L.P. (1985). *Psychology Research, Public Policy and Practice.* New York, NY: Praeger.

Kerns, L.L. & Bradley, W.J. (1990). Factors influencing psychiatric hospitalization. *EAP Digest,* Sept/Oct., 28–65.

Kiesler, C.A. (1991). U.S. mental health policy: Doomed to fail. Under editorial review.

Kiesler, C.A. & Morton, T.L. (1988). Prospective payment system for inpatient psychiatry: The advantages of controversy. *American Psychologist, 43,* 141–50.

Kiesler, C.A. & Sibulkin, A.E. (1987). *Mental Hospitalization: Myths and Facts about a National Crisis.* Newbury Park, CA: Sage Publishing, Inc.

Klerman, G.L. (1985). The role of the federal government in mental health services. In, Kasschau, R.A., Rehm, L.P., & Ullman, L.P. (Eds.), *Psychology Research, Public Policy and Practice.* New York, NY: Praeger.

Luborsky, L. Crits-Christoph, P., Mintz, J., & Auerbach, A. (1988). *Who will Benefit from Psychotherapy? Predicting Therapeutic Outcomes.* New York, NY: Basic Books, Inc.

Naditch, M.P. (1989). Measuring up: The dawning era of outcome management. *American Journal of Preventive Psychiatry & Neurology, 2:*1, Sept., 154–162.

Nguyen, T.D., Attkisson, C.C. & Stegner, B.L. (1983). Assessment of patient satisfaction:

Development and refinement of a service evaluation questionnaire. *Evaluation and Program Planning, 6,* 299–314.

Pallak, M.S. (1989). Defining and delivering effective and cost-effective mental health services. Invited address, Behavioral Healthcare Tomorrow Conference, Washington, D.C.

Pallak, M.S. & Cummings, N.A. (1992). Inpatient and outpatient psychiatric treatment: The effect of matching patients to appropriate levels of treatment on psychiatric and medical surgical hospital days. *Applied and Preventive Psychology: Current Scientific Perspectives, 1,* 83–87.

Pallak, M.S. & Kilburg, R.K. (1986). Psychology, public affairs and public policy: A strategy and review. *American Psychologist, 41,* 933–940.

Pallak, M.S., Cummings, N.A., Dörken, H.D., & Henke, C.J. (1991). The Impact of Psychological Intervention on Health Care Costs and Utilization: The Hawaii Medicaid Project. Contract Report No. 11-C-98344/9, HCFA.

Perloff, E. (1991). *Health and Psychosocial Instruments (HAPI).* Pittsburgh, PA: Behavioral Measurement Database Services.

Schlesinger, H., Mumford, E., Glass, G., Patrick, C. & Sharfstein, S. (1983). Mental health treatment and medical care utilization in a fee-for-service system: Outpatient mental health treatment following the onset of a chronic disease. *American Journal of Public Health, 73,* 422–429.

Smith, M., Glass, G.V. & Miller, T. (1980). *The Benefits of Psychotherapy.* Baltimore, MD: The Johns Hopkins University Press.

Stevens, R. (1989). *In Sickness and in Wealth: American Hospitals in the Twentieth Century.* New York, NY: Basic Books.

Ware, J.D. (1991). Measuring patient function and well-being: Some lessons from the medical outcomes study. In Heithoff, K. & Lohr, K. (Eds.), *Effectiveness and Outcomes in Health Care.* Washington, D.C.: National Academy Press.

Ware, J.E. & Sherbourne, C.D. (1991). *The SF-36 Short Form Health Status Survey: I. Conceptual Framework and Item Selection.* Boston, MA: New England Medical Centers Hospital, International Resource Center for Health Care Assessment.

RESOURCES

Health and Psychosocial Instruments (HAPI)
PO Box 110287
Pittsburgh, PA 15232-0787

InterStudy
PO Box 458
Excelsior, MN 55331-0458

International Resource Center for Health Care Assessment
NEMCH–Box 345
750 Washington Street
Boston, MA 02111

National Computer Systems, Inc.
5605 Green Circle Drive
Minnetonka, MN 55343

Strategic Advantage, Inc.
1484 Dupont Ave So.
Minneapolis, MN 55403

Chapter 13

EVALUATING PSYCHIATRIC AND SUBSTANCE ABUSE CASE MANAGEMENT ORGANIZATIONS

ARNOLD MILSTEIN, MARY HENDERSON, JEFFREY BERLANT, AND DONALD ANDERSON

The objective of mental health and chemical dependency case management organizations (CMOs) is to curb unnecessary services and inadequacies in quality of care. Primarily operating via phone contact with service providers before and during episodes of treatment, most of these companies are less than eight years old and have rarely been rigorously evaluated. There are four primary techniques by which case management organizations can be evaluated. Each technique has as a focus a different aspect of the services management process.

1. Direct evaluation of case management operations via on-site interviews and observation of a CMO's staff, and independent clinical assessment of their judgments and interventions via examination of staff work sheets.
2. Evaluation of claims data in order to gauge the impact of the CMO on service utilization and cost.
3. Evaluation of provider medical records for cases which have been subject to CMO scrutiny in order to assess the CMO's success in detecting and curbing unnecessary and poor quality services.
4. Evaluation of patient satisfaction with interactions with CMO staff as well as with care recommended by these staff.

This chapter focuses on the first two evaluation methods, because they are the most frequently utilized. We take a different approach in our discussion of each method. With respect to the first method—on-site operational evaluation—we describe the most common implementation problems observed during audits conducted by National Medical Audit/ Medical Audit Service (NMA) of William M. Mercer, Incorporated. The discussion is based on the results of 2–4 day on-site visits conducted in over 30 CMOs by the NMA audit team consisting of a clinical psychologist,

222

a board certified psychiatrist, and a registered nurse who is also a psychologist.

In the case of the second method—evaluation of claims data—we have focused on the critical steps necessary to increase the rigor of the data analysis and, thereby, the validity of the conclusions. We adopted this more conceptual focus because many of the claims-based evaluations which we have reviewed suffer from fundamental design failures. Accordingly, a review of common findings to date would have little meaning.

Evaluation via On-Site Operations Assessment

Three broad areas of the organization's functioning are examined during an audit: issues of access; utilization management and case management issues; and provider system issues (including networks and quality assurance programs directed at providers). The organization's own operating plan and the audit team's judgment of industry-wide "best practices" are used as dual frames of reference for the audit.

The site visit includes two components: (1) an examination of the documentation of the case management system, including direct review of case management records for recent inpatient and outpatient cases; and (2) "walking through a case," in which members of the audit team follow the management of specific cases from the time of the first phone call until the case is closed. The audits have revealed many common problems in organization and functioning across the CMOs visited.

Findings from Site Visits

Overall, there is great variation in how organizations are structured, how they do things, and what causes them problems. Some organizations which have successfully solved quite difficult problems in one area often have major unresolved problems in another. Very few organizations do everything badly, but no organization has achieved industry best practices in all dimensions. The following summary describes the most common deficiencies, grouped by the types of factors which the team evaluates during an audit.

PHONE SYSTEMS. Some programs which handle a high volume of cases do not have an automated call distribution system and, hence, a certain number of calls are "abandoned." The rate of abandoned calls generally ranges from 1% to 20%. Our standard for acceptable performance is an abandonment rate below 5%.

Many programs have a secretary or other non-clinician who answers the initial phone call from a patient. There is no inherent problem with this practice, as long as calls are ultimately directed to someone who is qualified to deal effectively with the problem at hand, and as long as the waiting time to reach the correct party is kept short. The skill of the person who answers the initial call is crucial in determining whether calls, which may involve complex clinical issues, are handled sensitively and are directed to an appropriately qualified case manager.

TRIAGE ISSUES. Every system should devise a mechanism for directing calls to case managers qualified to deal with the particular types of services being reviewed. Many systems, however, do not even attempt to address this problem and direct calls to case managers in a random fashion. The best referral systems have built-in mechanisms to ensure that calls get directed to the case managers whose capabilities are matched to the particular clinical issues. For example, cases with medication issues should be directed to a psychiatric nurse rather than a social worker. Similarly, substance abuse cases should be directed to case managers specifically qualified and experienced in this area.

Many systems have also ignored the problem of proper case matching when making referrals to therapists. In contrast, some systems are able to tailor referrals, based on considerations such as gender of the therapist, language and ethnicity requirements, and geographical convenience. For those benefit plans which cover a broad spectrum of mental health providers (e.g., M.D., Ph.D., M.S.W., R.N.), CMO's have yet to rise to the challenge of developing a practical theory for matching cases to provider credentials.

UTILIZATION REVIEW CRITERIA. Most organizations have criteria that specify clear behavioral indicators for levels of care. Some organizations, however, have adopted vague criteria which do not provide effective guidance to the case manager. Some organizations use published 50th percentile norms to assign initial length of stay, thus missing the opportunity to influence less severe cases for which discharge earlier than the 50th percentile norm would be achievable. Others use unmodified InterQual criteria (InterQual, 1992), which are insufficiently specific to effectively differentiate between conventional and optimally efficient care. A minority of organizations have refined their criteria to embody the following optimal characteristics: (1) age- and diagnosis-specific; (2) behaviorally descriptive; and (3) encompassing all levels of care, such as intensive day treatment and non-hospital residential care. Most, however, have detailed criteria only for acute inpatient care.

STAFF QUALIFICATIONS. Some organizations lack case managers or even supervisory personnel who have relevant mental health and substance abuse training and experience in both inpatient and outpatient settings. Some lack doctoral level reviewers who can engage in review as peers with doctoral level service providers. Some lack board certified psychiatrists for psychiatric review; others lack board certified child psychiatrists for child and adolescent cases or experienced chemical dependency (CD) specialists for substance abuse cases. One organization employed an internist without any psychiatric or CD experience as the psychiatric medical director. Although there is lingering controversy over the proper requirements for case managers—credentials or equivalent experience—some organizations have not made even a reasonable effort to ensure appropriate qualifications among their case management and review staff.

ORGANIZATION. CMOs vary significantly in the adequacy with which they define job descriptions and staff reporting relationships. There are also differences in the extent to which the structure of the organization is logical for the tasks to be performed. Sometimes responsibility for closely related tasks is lodged in different departments, or located on different floors of a building. This may result in poor communication between, for instance, the staff conducting patient intake and those responsible for reviewing, and in subsequent lengthy delays in initiating review.

Another common inadequacy is when ongoing management of a case is not formally assigned to a single reviewer. The result can be a "wheel of fortune" effect for follow-up reviews. The review is done by whichever reviewer is available, whether or not that reviewer is familiar with the case. This tends to result in lengthy delays while the reviewer peruses case notes, and in the loss of an opportunity for a case manager to build a positive working relationship with the provider.

INTERNAL QUALITY CONTROL PROGRAMS. Despite their tremendous importance for quality maintenance and improvement, internal quality control (QC) programs focused on the case management process are not comprehensive and are rarely rigorous. Some organizations have no discernible internal QC program, and many more have ineffective nominal systems at best. The following activities are fundamental to a QC program:

- Educationally oriented interdisciplinary conferences, such as clinical rounds.
- Regular direct observation and coaching of the case managers by clinically qualified supervisors.
- Routine internal clinical audits of case management notes which examine quality of judgment as well as adequacy of documentation.
- Tracking of staff-specific outcome data, adjusted for case mix.
- Inservice training programs shaped and driven by the findings of an internal QC monitoring system, including all of the above activities.

Inservice training seems to be a particular area of weakness in CMOs. Many organizations select inservice training programs arbitrarily or in response to staff requests for topics of interest rather than on the basis of assessed need. One audited program had a series of inservice training sessions directed toward non-mental health issues; another had no inservice training at all.

CLINICAL INFORMATION GATHERING. The best review organizations have developed on-line computer capability, employing a variety of management information systems to gather and summarize clinical data. Some, however, have stayed with paper-based systems. Few have advanced to the point where case managers engage in direct on-screen input of clinical information obtained during calls. Generally, organizations rely on delayed input of information recorded initially on paper forms.

Many of the on-line computerized systems which do exist have significant shortcomings. In some, there are lengthy delays when moving between screens or retrieving information from other sections. Other systems lack satisfactory word processing functions, resulting in hard-to-read, sometimes bizarre, records (e.g., "therapist" wrapping from one line to another as "the rapist").

Few CMOs have well-organized, systematic, logically constructed information gathering systems which effectively support decision-making at critical points. For example, few systems incorporate simple prompts to ensure that adequate clinical information is gathered and clear judgments made with respect to the absence or presence of medical necessity. Most have no type of classification system for quality of care problems such as misdiagnosis, improper prescribing practices, missed therapeutic opportunities, iatrogenic medication intoxications, inadequate mix and intensity of psychotherapeutic services, discharge planning errors, and management of concomitant medical problems.

Of special note is the universal absence of any provision for documenting suggestions and recommendations made to a provider about alternative approaches to treatment or level of care, and of provider responses to those recommendations. Though documentation of the clinical indicators for treatment is generally adequate, there tends to be very little documentation of case management activities. Physician advisors often claim that they frequently make quality of care recommendations to providers—and they no doubt do—but there is little documentation of what transpired. This information system deficit results in derivative deficits in internal quality control and risk management.

TIMELINESS OF REVIEW. Precertification is often the single most important intervention by a CMO, particularly in cases where an unnecessary inpatient admission with its concomitant social dislocations and life disruptions can be prevented. Across the audited programs, the percentage of cases in which precertification review actually precedes hospitalization ranges from 0% to about 60%. Most of the time this percentage is below 20%. This problem can be ascribed partly to poor employer education of employees (they are not aware of the necessity for precertification) and providers' failure to inform the CMO of an impending hospitalization. Still, however, there is evidence in a significant number of cases that initial notification was timely, but internal delays prevented certification prior to admission. Occasionally, individuals calling with preadmission notifications are told to call back after admission. Sometimes these cases are even reviewed after hospital discharge, due to lengthy internal processing delays.

No CMOs have designed and successfully implemented an effective system for promoting preadmission certifications, including an adequate educational program, designated qualified clinicians available for face-to-face preadmission clinical assessment, rapid processing of preadmission notifications, and systematic application of penalties for late notification. Few CMOs even have a place on their case management forms for recording that notification was late and that penalties should be applied.

As indicated above, substantial delays are common between initial notification by the provider and initial review. These average from one to as many as five days, depending on the system. Most often, delays are caused by inefficient document or information flow within the organization, and occasionally by ineffective systems for re-contacting providers. Good systems ensure same-day preadmission review, and concurrent review within one day of the initiation of treatment.

Continued stay reviews of a case (CSR) should occur at least every seven days; more frequent review should depend upon clinical circumstances. Initial CSR interviews, following the admission review, have averaged four to 13 days in various organizations. Most organizations do not satisfy their own standard for review intervals, which typically range from four to seven days but are sometimes as long as 14 days. The ideal of case-specific initial review intervals, tailored to the clinical circumstances, is seldom observed.

PHYSICIAN INVOLVEMENT. Delays in reviews by physician advisors for cases referred to them for a second opinion are significant in some systems. Average delays range from one day to five days. Given the importance of rapid response to cases identified as urgent and needing higher levels of attention, delays beyond one day are undesirable. Sometimes such a delay is due to the lack of easy access to the proper physician advisor (for instance, a child psychiatrist for an adolescent case). Certainly in those systems with no in-house physician reviewers, especially subspecialty reviewers, delays can be expected. Sometimes, however, there are delays in response even in systems which do have in-house physician advisors. The reasons for this can be obscure. In well-functioning systems, physician advisors are involved in the routine supervision of the case management function. Ready case manager access to physicians and informal discussion of difficult cases is absent from some systems, to their detriment.

Physician advisor training programs and quality control efforts targeted at physician advisors are seldom found. The presence of a full-time or near full-time medical director can improve the reliability and consistency of physician advisor responses, but only if the need for quality control of physician advisor decisions is recognized. Peer review of physician advisor decisions is rarely present, but is always needed.

MEDICAL NECESSITY DETERMINATIONS. All cases reviewed by our on-site assessment team are subjected to an independent assessment by a physician team member to determine medical necessity based on the information available in the case management record. In some instances, inadequate documentation of the clinical picture makes this assessment difficult. Direct observation of the case managers as they conduct reviews helps to corroborate findings from the case records.

Medically unnecessary admissions, which currently constitute between

10% and 30% of private insurance cases, are detected and acted upon by CMOs to differing extents. Many organizations are unable to recognize and curb these unnecessary admissions.

Evidence is not often present that case decisions were made in accordance with the organization's official utilization criteria set. At the same time, some review criteria are so vague as to give little practical direction to the reviewers' activities. It is not uncommon for reviewers and physician advisors to create their own informal set of rules which may not always correspond to the CMO's written criteria.

Some systems exhibit a lack of clarity regarding the review decision and communication of this decision to the provider. Sometimes evidence of a distinct review event—with a clear beginning, middle, and end—cannot be found in the documentation. Sometimes the specific type or quantity of care which was approved cannot be determined from the documents. Cases which are referred for physician advisor review and subsequently reviewed after some period of delay frequently lack a clear statement about what was finally approved. Even in systems with adequate documentation of decisions, a clear message may not have been given verbally to the provider by the case manager.

QUALITY OF CARE PROBLEM IDENTIFICATION. Independent review of CMO clinical records indicates that these organizations typically fail to recognize half of the quality of care problems for which there is evidence. Sometimes none of the problems appear to have been detected. Of those which are recognized, only about half are referred to the physician and then acknowledged or acted upon by the advisor. Physician advisors claim that they routinely deal with quality problems but rarely document their actions. At best, then, documentation of this important function is lacking. It appears that all CMOs could benefit significantly from improvements in the identification of quality problems and systematic efforts to correct them.

Evaluating CMOs by Analyzing Claims Data: A Stepwise Path

There are six critical steps in the process of evaluating the effectiveness of case management programs using health care claims data:

1. Specifying the question or questions to be addressed by the analysis.
2. Determining the strongest and most efficient study design.
3. Defining the outcome measures.

4. Selecting the data base.
5. Identifying the groups (and subgroups) for analysis.
6. Performing the analysis.

In this section of the chapter, key components of each of these steps are described. It should be stressed that claims data have significant limitations as a source of information about the quality and cost-effectiveness of care rendered to mental health/chemical dependency patients. Nevertheless, they represent a readily available and relatively inexpensive data repository which usually spans several years of experience for the population of interest. Furthermore, the quality and comprehensiveness of claims data, particularly for outpatient care, have significantly improved in recent years, a trend that will doubtless continue due to unceasing pressure from government and private payers for more accurate information about claimants' treatment experiences.

Step 1: Specifying the Questions

An often overlooked step in the evaluation process is the specification of the question or questions to be answered by the analysis. When using claims data, this is particularly important, because many relevant or interesting questions may not be answerable due to data limitations. For example, one may wish to determine if the patients selected for case management have the same level of severity of illness or functional status limitations as those in the group not selected by the program. Since limited clinical information is available in claims data, questions of this type cannot be adequately addressed and thus should not be considered the major focus of study.

When developing the questions to be addressed, the evaluator must consider who are the consumers of the evaluation results and what they most need to know about the case management program. For example, is the consumer an employer deciding whether or not a mental health/ chemical dependency case management program should be instituted? Is the consumer an insurer or an employer who wishes to know if the case management program is working effectively? Is the consumer a case management program which wants to find out if it is targeting the services most in need of case management?

A final consideration relates to the goals of the case management program itself. In evaluating effectiveness, it is important to know if the program is focusing primarily on controlling costs, improving quality of care, or both. Does the program concern itself with only mental health and chemical dependency claims or does it also focus on treatment of medical conditions which are sequelae of or otherwise related to psychological or chemical dependency problems (e.g., anorexia nervosa, cirrhosis)?

Examples of questions that often can be adequately addressed by health care claims data are as follows:

- Does the case management program lower per claimant cost outlays for mental health/chemical dependency services?
- Does the case management program lower per claimant total health care expenditures?
- Does the case management program shorten inpatient lengths of stay?
- Does the case management program negotiate lower fees with providers?
- Does the case management program improve continuity of care?
- Does the case management program improve patient access to alternative services?
- Is the case management program focusing on the types of cases which would benefit most from case management?
- For which conditions is the case management program particularly effective and for which is it relatively ineffective?
- Are case managed patients more likely than others to experience patterns of care which are in accordance with best practice models?

The first six questions can be addressed by claims data alone. The last three questions require linking the claims data with information from the case management program. Analysis of claims data with regard to case management requires knowledge of which patients were subject to this process. The CMO needs to identify these patients using a unique number which is common to the claims file (e.g., social security number or employee number).

It should be noted that care must be taken when using employee number for this purpose, since often this number is used by the insurance company both for the employee and for his or her dependents. The employee number, therefore, should be used as an identifier only in conjunction with another variable, such as first name, birth date, or position in family.

Step 2: Determining the Study Design

Determining the strongest and yet the most efficient study design is the most crucial step in the study. The goal of this process is to maximize the validity of the study. A study is valid if the conclusions drawn from its results are true, within acceptable statistical margins of error.

Implicit in most of the questions listed above is the corresponding question: Would similar results have been obtained in the absence of the case management program? The most scientifically valid way of determining this is to use a true experimental design with random assignment to conditions. In this design, one group of patients would be randomly assigned to the case management program while another group of patients would be randomly assigned to a regular care group. While random assignment has been employed in some major health services research projects (for example, the RAND health insurance experiment [Manning, 1984]), this is not a practical approach for most evaluation research. Therefore, alternative approaches must be considered. Information about and hypothetical data from four alternative designs are presented in Table 1.

The weakest design, which is unfortunately employed all too often in health care evaluation, is the *one-group case study design* (Design 1, Table 1). If such a design is used to evaluate the impact of a case management program, only the experience of the case managed group is measured and it is measured at one point in time. In the example in Table 1, the analysis revealed that case managed patients averaged 6.7 admissions per year per thousand plan members for mental health and chemical dependency services, and the per admission total charge averaged approximately $7,000. Unfortunately, without a benchmark to use for comparison purposes, these data are not interpretable. Comparing the results to national or industry-wide averages is usually not appropriate since the casemix (type, frequency, and severity of diagnoses within the sample), other characteristics of the group of interest, or the benefit design are likely to be significantly different from the national or industry-wide groups. The best use of such data may be as baseline for investigating change, as is discussed below.

The second design which is often used is the *pre-test, post-test one group design* (Design 2, Table 1). In this approach, the experience of the case managed group is measured before the implementation of the program and again after the program has been operating for a specified period of

Table 1

Information Yielded by Four Study Designs

Results

Design	Measure	Case-Managed Group		Comparison Group		Conclusion
		Pre	Post	Pre	Post	
1. One group case study	Admissions per 1000 members		6.7			Uninterpretable
	Payment per admission		$7,000			
2. Pre-test, post-test	Admissions per 1000 members	9.0	6.7			Case management controls utilization and cost
	Payment per admission	$13,000	$7,000			
3. Comparison groups	Admissions per 1000 members		6.7		7.0	No sig. difference between managed and non-managed patients
	Payment per admission		$7,000		$7,200	
4. Pre-test, post-test comparison groups	Admissions per 1000 members	9.0	6.7	6.9	7.0	Case management controls the rate of increase in cost and utilization
	Payment per admission	$13,000	$7,000	$7,300	$7,200	

time. To continue the example above, the pre-test measure of the group showed that, before implementation of the program, mental health/ chemical dependency patients average 9.0 admissions per year per thousand plan members, and the total paid claims per episode of care averaged $13,000 (measured in constant dollars). The conclusion drawn from these results would probably be that case management is highly effective in controlling costs and utilization. The factor which threatens the validity of this conclusion, however, is *history*. That is, events other than implementation of a case management program could have caused changes in costs and utilization. For example, one company experienced a significant increase in mental health service utilization during a year in which the company was reorganized and many of its employees were relocated to different parts of the country.

A commonly used quasi-experimental design (Campbell & Stanley, 1966) is known as the *comparison group design* (Design 3, Table 1). Here, the experience of a group which is similar in selected measurable respects to the group in question (in this case, the case managed group) is chosen for comparison purposes and measured on the variables of interest in the study. Both the case managed group and the comparison group (whose care is not managed) are measured at only one point in time, after case management has been in operation for a specified period. For this application, the comparison group should have similar diagnostic, age, gender, employment and geographic distributions. Further, the benefit plans should be comparable.

To continue with the example in Table 1, measurement of the experience of the comparison group shows that mental health and chemical dependency patients averaged 7.0 admissions per year per thousand enrollees and had total paid claims per episode of care averaging $7,200 per patient, results very similar to those obtained for the case managed group. These results would likely lead one to conclude that case management has a small, but not significant (as demonstrated by statistical analysis), positive effect in controlling cost and utilization.

While the comparison group design is relatively strong, there are still threats to its validity. The major factor which poses the threat in this case is *selection* of the comparison group. That is, it is not always possible to know which variables should be used for matching the groups. If critical variables are not controlled, the comparison group ends up being not truly comparable for purposes of the analysis. For example, it has been observed that young, upwardly-mobile white collar employees tend not to utilize their mental health or chemical dependency benefits even if they consume such services. They prefer to pay for treatment themselves rather than risk their employer finding out that they have a behavioral health problem. A plan with a high percentage of such employees would tend to have relatively low utilization statistics.

The recommended approach is to use the strongest quasi-experimental design, the *pre-test, post-test, comparison group design* (Design 4, Table 1). It should be noted, however, that this design is the most expensive since it requires measurements at two different times for two groups of people: both the case managed and the comparison groups, before and after the implementation of the program. The advantage of this design is that it controls for both selection and history. In the example in Table 1, measurement of the comparison group before program implementation shows that the average number of admissions experienced by the comparison group was 6.9 per thousand enrollees and the average payments were $7,300 per episode of care. Analysis of these results would lead to the conclusion that case management is effective in controlling costs and utilization, since the rate of decrease in the case-managed group was greater than that in the comparison group.

Step 3: Defining Outcome Measures

Implicit in the selection of the evaluation question(s) to be addressed is the choice of variables to be used as outcome measures. For the evaluation of the effectiveness of a mental health/chemical dependency case management program, outcome measures will most commonly be defined in two domains: cost/utilization and quality/access.

Examples of cost/utilization outcomes include the following:

- mental health/chemical dependency services charged and paid amounts per claimant and per covered individual;
- total (for all health services) charged and paid amounts per claimant and per covered individual;
- inpatient admissions for mental health/chemical dependency per claimant and per covered individual;
- total inpatient admissions per claimant and per covered individual;
- average length of stay for mental health/chemical dependency admissions;

- mental health/chemical dependency outpatient visits per claimant and per individual;
- total outpatient visits per claimant and per covered individual;
- ratio of mental health/chemical dependency outpatient to inpatient total charged and paid amounts per claimant and per individual, and
- ratio of outpatient to inpatient total charged and paid amounts per claimant and per individual.

Quality and access issues are very difficult to address using claims data because of the paucity of clinical information generally available. The examples below are possible indicators of poor quality of care which may suggest the need for further investigation:

- different mental health/chemical dependency providers per claimant;
- total and per patient mental health/chemical dependency inpatient discharges not followed by outpatient care within two weeks;
- total and per patient mental health/chemical dependency readmissions within three months;
- total and per patient mental health/chemical dependency readmissions not preceded by outpatient care;
- total and per patient mental health/chemical dependency admissions exceeding a specific percentile (e.g., the 75th or 90th) for length of stay for the same DRG, as reported for national Blue Cross/Blue Shield data; and
- total and per patient mental health/chemical dependency admissions with length of stay less than three days.

Step 4: Selecting the Database

There are four major considerations related to the use of a claims database for the types of evaluation discussed here: size, time period covered by the data, unit of analysis, and database preparation.

SIZE. The claims database must yield a sufficient number of mental health/chemical dependency inpatient and outpatient claims to allow a reliable examination of patterns of care. Ideally, there should be at least 1,000 admissions for each group studied. Assuming a utilization rate of .10 (10% of covered individuals utilize services) and a ratio of mental health/chemical dependency admissions to total admissions of .05 (5% of utilizers receive treatment for mental health or substance dependence problems), the claims database for each group in the study should include 200,000 covered, or insured, individuals. Although use of smaller databases is feasible, an analysis (referred to as a "power" analysis) should always be carried out first to determine the minimum size group needed to detect a significant difference using the type of statistical tests chosen for the analysis.

TIME PERIOD. Both the incurred (when the service was provided) and the paid dates need to be considered when analyzing claims data, since there can be a long lag between these two events, particularly for claims of large dollar amounts. When specifying the time interval for the study, allowance must be made for the fact that, for the beginning point, the incurred and paid dates may be quite different. The paid date is usually designated as occurring within four to six months after the incurred date. The use of this claims "run-out" period ensures that virtually all the final payment amounts for claims incurred during the period of interest will be on the file.

The time period for the analysis will depend upon the design chosen for the study. For designs 1 and 3 in Table 1, only one time period is required. Generally, at least 12 months of claims data are included in such a study. Therefore, for a study investigating the impact of a case management program in 1989, the data set would include cases for which any claim was incurred between January 1, 1989 and December 31, 1989 (inclusive), and for which payment was made after January 1, 1989 but on or before June 30, 1990.

When using a pre-test, post-test design (designs 2 and 4 in Table 1), two time periods need to be selected. The pre-test period should be the 12-month period directly preceding the implementation of the program. To assure a more accurate measurement of the impact of the fully implemented case management program and to mitigate start-up effects, the post-test period should begin at least six months after program implementation. If fewer than 12 months are used for periods of analysis, the months included should be the same in both periods to avoid possible effects of seasonal variations.

UNIT OF ANALYSIS. The most appropriate unit of analysis for studying the impact of mental health/chemical dependency case management programs is the individual claimant rather than the admission or episode of care. This is because case management is designed to consider both the inpatient and outpatient experiences of individuals. Thus, claims should be aggregated over each individual claimant using a unique identifier. For selected analyses which focus on characteristics of the inpatient admission such as length of stay or number of different providers involved in the episode, the inpatient admission should be used as the unit of analysis. For analyses focusing on characteristics of outpatient care (number of sessions, frequency) the episode of care should be the unit of analysis.

DATABASE PREPARATION. Each claims database has unique features which must be understood and addressed for accurate interpretation of the results of analysis. At a minimum, the following determinations must be made prior to analysis:

- how claims adjustments will be handled;
- how interim claims (for which a treatment episode is not completed) will be analyzed;
- which claims are to be excluded from the analysis (e.g., Medicare claims or "coordination of benefits" in which the cost of services is shared by two different insurance programs); and
- how to account for co-payments and deductibles.

If claims files from different carriers, or even files from the same carrier representing different time periods, are to be combined, the data must be "standardized" before analysis. Issues to be considered here include:

- how to adjust for differences in coding practices for diagnoses or procedures;
- how to adjust for inflation claims from different time periods; and
- how to deal with changes in the Diagnosis Related Groups (DRG) grouper, if they are relevant to the analysis.

Sufficient time should be allocated to building the data files and testing the data base before the study is actually begun and before analysis commences.

Step 5: Identifying Groups and Subgroups for Analysis

A substantial portion of the analysis of the effectiveness of case management for mental health/chemical dependency will focus on patients who have experienced one or more inpatient admissions for this type of care. If a person-based file is being used, the group can be divided into those who were admitted with a primary diagnosis of a psychiatric or substance abuse disorder during the study period(s) and those who were not. For an admission-based file, admissions can be similarly divided.

A study by Goldstein, Bassuck et al. (1988) provides an example in which certain groups were excluded from the analysis because of the special circumstances related to their characteristics or their treatment. These groups included children under age 13 years and persons admitted for treatment of mental retardation. Adolescents (over age 13) with psychiatric diagnoses such as dysthymia and major affective disorder were grouped into the appropriate diagnostic category and treated as other members of the sample. The authors defined a special subgroup, designated "adolescent nonpsychotic," which included diagnoses of conduct disorders, attention deficit disorders, and anxiety disorders of adolescence. Experience shows that this group is likely to account for a significant portion of mental health/chemical dependency admissions and that lengths of stay and treatment costs for these admissions are likely to be relatively high. Effects of a case management activity may be quite marked in cases of this type. Therefore, this group was singled out for special attention in the analysis of the effectiveness of the case management organization.

Step 6: Analyzing the Data

Once the analytical file is created, descriptive statistics on the sample characteristics and the selected outcome measures can be calculated for each group defined in the study design. Sample characteristics should be analyzed to describe the groups as well as to confirm that groups which are supposed to be comparable are actually similar on important variables. Diagnosis, age, gender, treatment setting (e.g., general hospital, free-standing psychiatric hospital, alcohol/chemical dependency treatment center), and location are the most important sample characteristics to analyze.

Differences among study groups on both sample characteristics and outcome variables (e.g., average mental health/chemical dependency treatment charges/payments, average number of mental health/chemical dependency admissions, average number of different mental health/chemical dependency providers) can be analyzed using the appropriate statistical tests of significance. The most commonly used are the chi-square test for *categorical* variables (e.g., when looking at differences in numbers of males versus females across groups), and analysis of variance for *interval* variables (e.g., when comparing two groups on total payments). More complex *multi-variate* analyses such as ordinary least squares regression and logistic regression can be used to examine the relative effects of a group of variables or for determining the impact of a single variable—case management—while holding all other variables constant.

CONCLUSION

Despite the large market share enjoyed by mental health and chemical dependency case management organizations, these are still early days in the development of large scale case review and case management programs. Close inspection of the CMOs indicates great variation in both structure and process. Variation is to be expected in a young industry, particularly in one which has grown as rapidly as managed care, but it is also the enemy of quality.

While each CMO has its own strengths, each also has significant weaknesses, many of which, as has been seen, are quite apparent to the external observer. As long as these weaknesses go uncorrected case management organizations are vulnerable to the continuing criticisms of providers, consumers, and advocates. There are no accepted standards and little regulation which currently apply to managed care organizations. An obvious question, then, is whether the industry should embark upon a program of self-regulation or self-monitoring which would provide some assurance of adherence to minimal standards of performance on the part of case management organizations. Accepting such a challenge would signal the beginnings of maturity in the managed care industry.

REFERENCES

Campbell, D.T., & Stanley, J.C. (1966). *Experimental and Quasi-Experimental Designs for Research.* Chicago: Rand-McNally.

Goldstein, J.M., Bassuck, E., Holland, S., & Zimmer, D. (1988). Identifying Catastrophic Psychiatric Cases. *Medical Care, 26,* 790–799.

InterQual (1992). *The ISD-A™ Review System with ISD-A™ Criteria.* North Hampton, NH: InterQual.

Manning, W.G. (1984). A controlled trial of the effect of a prepaid group practice on use of services. *New England Journal of Medicine, 310,* 1505–1510.

PART VII
CONSTRUCTING THE FUTURE

Chapter 14

THE WAY AHEAD: THE PROMISE AND CHALLENGES OF MANAGED BEHAVIORAL HEALTH CARE

SHARON A. SHUEMAN, WARWICK G. TROY AND SAMUEL L. MAYHUGH

T he most common argument put forth by critics of managed care asserts that the cost concerns of these companies inevitably result in compromises to quality. Implicit in this argument is that the quality of traditional fee-for-service care is the standard, despite the fact no empirical evidence supports the contention that the quality of behavioral health services provided under traditional payment structures exceeds that for managed services. In fact, much anecdotal evidence has been offered to support the opposite position. Further, prior to the advent of managed care as a burgeoning industry, little interest had been expressed in issues of quality by either providers or sanctioners.

Few, if any, of the characteristics of traditional fee-for-service systems could be said to advance quality of services. In contrast, a number of elements in the design of managed care programs do suggest a potential for both quality improvement and cost saving. This chapter focuses on those aspects of managed programs which are judged to have significant promise for contributing positively to cost containment and quality of behavioral health services. While companies will, of course, vary greatly in their capacity to exploit these aspects, the core characteristics of these systems provide an adequate foundation for every company to contribute in some way to improvements in the quality of services provided.

The promise of managed care can only be realized, however, if the industry is able to deal effectively with major challenges which confront it. The challenges discussed in the latter part of the chapter are of two types: (1) *developmental,* reflecting the kind of quality control problems inevitably arising within innovative or rapidly developing programs; and (2) *structural,* which must be dealt with through collaborative efforts such as between the managed care industry and governments, training programs, and provider communities. The developmental problems would be expected to diminish as the managed care industry matures, assuming these companies take seriously their responsibilities for accountability to consumers, employers, and providers. One can be less sanguine, however, about the capacity of the industry to forge the alliances and put forth the considerable effort required to respond successfully to the more complex structural challenges. Only if this occurs will managed care truly come into its own as a uniquely American arrangement (Rodriguez, 1989) incorporating both funding and service delivery within a single entity.

THE PROMISE OF MANAGED SYSTEMS

Despite the problems apparent in their implementation, managed models of service delivery would seem to have much to offer. In stark contrast to traditional service delivery programs—most typically fee-for-service—managed programs are characterized by two elements which are fundamental to their success: they incorporate a *service system*, and they provide a *level of control* necessary to assess and improve quality. In addition, by their very nature, managed care programs manifest the necessity for accountability by providers to external sanctioners.

The systematic approach of managed care facilitated by the information technology common to such systems can usefully illuminate service delivery, resulting in a better understanding of the clinical process, what works and what does not, at what cost, and which providers appear to be more effective than others. This increased "intelligence" combined with greater control gives managed systems the capacity to design and implement quality assessment and improvement activities not possible in non-managed programs.

Promise: Increased Understanding of the Clinical Situation

The monitoring and information management capabilities of managed systems have "opened up" the previously sacrosanct clinical relationship, allowing the collection of more precisely targeted clinical data on treatment processes and their effects on specific disorders. At the individual case level, such information provides the justification for intervention by the case manager to improve the quality of care. In the aggregate, these kinds of data constitute the basis for establishing process-outcome links and developing and modifying practice guidelines, the validation of which can ultimately lead to more effective treatments when promulgated as intervention protocols.

The use of clinical data to develop provider profiles presents opportunities for determining the relative strengths and weakness of various provider (disciplinary) groups with regard to particular constellations of patients or problems. Managed systems are able, therefore, to make better use of practitioner groups by articulating for them specific roles based on evaluations of cost-effectiveness across a range of treatment situations. In the interest of beneficiaries, these systems can also promote collaboration and referral among practitioner groups within a network by delineating interdisciplinary referral criteria and procedures.

Provider profiling also allows a determination, from an outcome perspective, of some of the weaknesses in professional training programs. Such evidence can constitute a basis for discussions between managed care companies and training programs which might, ultimately, result in changes to established academic training practices and to collaborative training activities. Profiling can also be used in the design of supplementary training and professional development programs conducted independently within the managed care industry.

Promise: Increased Efficacy in Comprehensive Service Systems

No large, managed medical-surgical system can reasonably claim to offer a comprehensive and effective system of health and medical care in the absence of a behavioral health program integrated within the larger system of care. Some unique contributions of a managed behavioral health component to the effectiveness of a larger general health care entity are as follows: identification of beneficiaries whose pattern of medical services utilization suggests a possible need for referral for behavioral health services, such as was done so successfully within the Kaiser-Permanente program (Follette & Cummings, 1967); targeting of patients whose medical conditions are exacerbated by problems which are amenable to behavioral intervention (for example, patients suffering from high blood pressure, diabetes, or other physical conditions aggravated by maladaptive lifestyles); and identification of patients whose apparent emotional problems may have a medical cause (such as may be true for certain conditions presenting as anxiety disorders).

Promise: Improved Accessibility to and Appropriateness of Services

A properly implemented managed care process allows the case manager, in consultation with the provider, to develop a treatment plan appropriate for the patient, without regard to the limitations and prohibitions inherent in traditional benefit plans. This is known as having a "flexible benefit." Under traditional fee-for-service plans, for example, it was not uncommon for day treatment programs or other less costly alternatives to acute inpatient care to be disallowed, despite their cost advantage and their appropriateness as treatment options in particular instances. Such endemic inflexibility resulted in providers exaggerating the severity of a patient's problems to prevent discharge to the only allowed alternative— outpatient therapy. Under managed systems, providers have far less incentive, other than a financial one, to misrepresent aspects of the case to justify continuation of a particular type of treatment. In the better managed systems, case managers have the authority to provide access to a service exclusively on the basis of its appropriateness rather than its service category, cost, or location. Through their extensive knowledge of service options, case managers may also be able to identify and access particular resources of which the direct service provider is unaware.

Creating More Appropriate Benefit Plans. Flexible managed programs give employers maximum latitude in determining the objectives of the particular benefit plan they pay for. For example, under traditional plans, interventions such as marital counseling were often not covered since the targets of such interventions, in this case marital problems, were not considered "diagnosable mental illness." Given that marital problems in and of themselves can have negative consequences on an employee's work performance, providing coverage for focused, strategic marital counseling may be a cost-effective option for an employer in the medium to long term. The better managed care plans permit employers to decide what they want to achieve with a benefit plan and, with the help of the managed care company, design an appropriate benefit structure and service network to realize the desired service objectives.

THE CHALLENGES TO MANAGED SYSTEMS

Juxtaposed with the significant promise of managed care are a set of bedeviling challenges to this developing industry. While these challenges do not threaten the immediate survival of managed health care—indeed, there appears to be no reasonable alternative to this approach—they do have the capacity to seriously limit the extent to which managed systems will be able to accomplish their service cost and quality objectives while recognizing the needs and concerns of consumers, employers, and providers.

Challenge: To Reduce Variation in the Quality of Managed Systems

Evidence from formal evaluations of managed care companies (Milstein, Henderson, Berlant, & Anderson, 1994) indicates that the quality of these programs varies greatly across the industry. In some instances, it would appear, these companies fail to maintain a level of quality equivalent to that which they demand from their own network service providers.

There is an obvious need for the development and implementation of appropriate company-wide training programs, processes for monitoring and supervision of staff, and evaluation activities to ensure that a company's policies are reasonable, that case management services are appropriate, acceptable to providers, and delivered with consistency, that they accurately reflect established policies, and that case management and review personnel are competent. Competence is a particularly critical issue, since a perceived lack of competence among case management personnel has had a significant negative impact on the credibility of case management organizations and on the willingness of providers to comply with their accountability requirements.

Challenge: To Achieve Uniformity in Critical Policies

There is a conspicuous lack of uniformity across managed care programs with regard to critical policies such as scope and content of practice guidelines, information requirements for treatment plans, and criteria for determining necessity of care. Such differences are unnecessarily confusing and burdensome and provide significant obstacles for providers who make genuine attempts to conduct their practices according to the basic tenets of good quality care—tenets reflecting a "higher truth" which should transcend programs. Industry-wide efforts, some supported by initiatives of government or other funding organizations, the mental health professions, and the research community, will be required to reach consensus on certain policies central to managed care. Consensus efforts will only occur, however, if participants in the managed care industry genuinely perceive such an objective as benefiting the industry rather than compromising their particular company's competitive position.

INDUSTRY ACCREDITATION. It has been argued that a voluntary accreditation program would solve some of the problems of the managed care industry, including inadequate training of review and case management personnel, inconsistency in policies across companies, and variability in the implementation of policies. While formal accreditation programs have not been demonstrated to contribute significantly to quality of outcome in health and human services, they do provide the consumer with some assurance that a program's policies and procedures are consistent with minimum standards agreed to and supported by the industry itself. Given the significant variability across managed programs, there is little doubt that even such an essentially mechanistic approach to the implementation of minimum standards would, in due course, lift the overall level of quality within the industry. Participation in the institutional self-study process as part of voluntary accreditation has been associated with modest improvements in the organizational "climate" of services provision. Importantly, in view of the competitive nature of the industry, a formal accreditation effort would probably be enthusiastically embraced by managed care companies, if only for marketing purposes.

Challenge: To Integrate Providers into Managed Systems

The adversarial nature of the relationship between managed care programs and providers is perhaps the most pervasive problem besetting the managed care industry. The prolongation of this state of affairs is very likely to have disturbingly negative consequences for the quality of individual clinical interventions and, consequently, for the health status of beneficiaries. Ultimately, it will affect the quality of the service systems. It will also effectively prevent providers from assuming an appropriate role in the shaping of managed care programs.

It is axiomatic that the quality of services can neither be assessed nor improved without the cooperation of major stakeholder groups. Until providers and programs do a better job of working together in the interest of all parties, the case management process will remain haphazard and its efficacy unacceptably variable. Better quality control of the case management process as well as the establishment of consensus policies will obviously make working with managed programs less problematic for providers. Any such developments, however, will not ultimately resolve the problems between providers and programs until provider networks are more effectively integrated into managed care companies. This, in turn, is not likely to occur as long as providers continue to be able to contract with multiple case management organizations, functioning as traditional independent practitioners with merely an "overlay" of case management. This is a particular structural problem which attacks the very basis of quality improvement.

CREATING TRUE SYSTEMS. Herein, then, lies perhaps the biggest immediate challenge for managed care companies: to make true systems out of the opportunistic and pragmatically devised arrangements which are now the rule rather than the exception for many programs. In true systems individual providers operate as part of an integrated group. They are in close proximity to professional peers with whom they regularly and freely consult, to whom they refer when appropriate, and from whom they receive referrals. They have a responsibility for providing all necessary services for the population of a specific "catchment area." They assume some financial risk for the services to the population but also receive financial or other incentives for improving service quality. Importantly, however, in this idealized vignette, providers are also given continuous access to services utilization data and individual feedback, and are guided by clear service policies, practice standards, and clinical protocols.

Clearly, such an arrangement would be difficult to replicate within the typical managed care context, if only because the employer focus of most benefit plans precludes implementation of a local "catchment area" arrangement. There are things, however, which managed programs can do to increase the coherence of the provider network and facilitate providers' identification with the managed system. The following are examples of operational policies which are designed to achieve this goal.

- Give preference in recruitment to professionals involved in group practices, particularly groups which possess established accountability systems.
- Limit the number of providers in the network in order to increase the volume of referrals which any provider receives from the single program. Do this by a careful process of selection and monitoring to identify and retain the most competent providers.
- Give the most competent providers a special designation (e.g., "quality assured"), and relieve them from at least some of the basal

administrative or accountability requirements of the case management process.

- Give these same providers increased responsibility in the system, for example, for orienting, consulting with, monitoring, and supporting new providers.
- Keep providers well informed about system policies and operations (e.g., through a periodic newsletter) and actively solicit their suggestions about policies and procedures.
- Provide a mix of financial incentives (for example, require no discounting of fees for "quality assured" providers).

Challenge: To Prepare Providers for Participation in Managed Systems

Managed care has created a drastically different practice environment from the one which most clinical practitioners have been prepared for by their education and training. The greatest difficulties in adjusting to managed care are experienced by providers practicing currently who are being asked to change both attitudes and behaviors "midstream" in their career. The first, most immediate challenges for managed care systems are to give these providers the support and assistance necessary to make the changes in their practice patterns and to actively and consistently engage these same providers in building better systems.

The other major challenge is one which must be confronted via collaborative efforts of managed care companies and graduate training programs, including psychiatry, psychology, and clinical social work. Training programs must, first and foremost, acknowledge the importance of managed service systems in behavioral health service provision. And, given the historical and prevailing isolation of programs from the world of practice, this is to ask a great deal. In academic contexts this is usually signified by the subject being treated as a formal course offering, whether field- or classroom-based. Students would not be expected to attain mastery of the relevant skills or concepts, but they should, as a result of their training experience, develop a basic understanding and acceptance of this mode of service delivery. Actual mastery would require a graduated sequence of formal post-degree experiences, monitoring, and collegial review for which managed companies ultimately need to take significant responsibility.

Challenge: To Implement Meaningful Research and Evaluation Activities

It is inevitable that within managed care increasing use will be made of research and evaluation mechanisms to assess all aspects of the impact of the service management process. While there is little doubt that the frequency of these kinds of activities will increase, there is significant uncertainty about the rigor and objectivity of such efforts, as well as the extent to which their findings will be made available to a non-proprietary audience for use in efforts to improve managed systems within the industry at large.

The competitive environment prevailing in health care would not be expected to foster the large-scale, multi-program research and evaluation ventures which would be of greatest benefit to the wider health services system. To ensure this objective, governments or foundations could usefully consider a greater commitment to providing funding for studies which transcend the unique interests of individual managed care programs. For these efforts to be meaningful, however, the managed care industry will itself need to adopt a less grudging public accountability stance and cooperate actively with organizations conducting such research. Participation by a cross section of the industry will provide a basis for examining — at a "macro" level — the effects of the various managed care models on critical behavioral health outcome indicators such as cost and quality of care; utilization patterns; and beneficiary, employer, and provider satisfaction.

Challenge: To Adopt a Genuine Commitment to Quality

Despite frequent public statements to the contrary, the commitment to quality of services within some managed care companies is inconsistent, with quality being seen by some managers primarily as a marketing tool. Assessing and improving the quality of clinical services, as well as that of the services management system, are complex tasks requiring sustained effort and a significant investment of resources. Furthermore, there is no guarantee that these investments will bring tangible benefits to the organization, beyond what could be achieved with effective marketing of inadequate quality management activities — particularly in the shorter term. There is no doubt that some companies will continue merely to pay lip service to the importance of quality assessment and management until there is incontrovertible evidence for the positive cost-benefit of such accountability mechanisms within managed care settings.

Challenge: To Improve Management and Utilization of Data

Managed care programs can not effectively manage their own systems, let alone the clinical services provided through their networks, without access to adequate computer-based management information systems (MIS). Furthermore, without a finely tuned MIS to support them, quality assurance activities as well as research and program evaluation efforts are so restricted as to be virtually useless.

The managed care industry has, by and large, not adequately exploited the potential of automated data management systems, although this may well be the area of greatest progress over the coming three to five years. In many cases, data systems currently used in managed programs are merely modified claims systems, yielding little more than a basic clinical data set (diagnosis, procedure code, amount of service) and information required for payment. Their capacity to increase, for example, a firm's understanding of the clinical process or to ensure consistency in the application of policies is minimal; as a consequence, they can do little to enhance the effectiveness of the case management process. It must be accepted as axiomatic that the capabilities of managed care systems will not advance without corresponding advances in the capabilities of MIS implemented within these systems.

Challenge: To Sustain Employer-Managed Care Contracts

A significant disadvantage from an accountability perspective is the lack of continuity in relationships between managed care companies and employers. All too often an employer will enter a contract for care management with a particular company, only to terminate that contract within two or three years due to lack of satisfaction with the service or wavering confidence in the company's capacity to deliver on its promises.

Failure to sustain contracted relationships makes it difficult, if not impossible, for the employer to answer the critical longer-term questions about the effect of behavioral health services on factors such as utilization of medical-surgical services or employee performance measures including absenteeism, job tenure, and incidence and consequences of industrial accidents. The prevalence of short-term arrangements also drastically limits the benefit of any illness prevention and health promotion program that may have been developed.

In this context, then, it is next to impossible for managed care companies to evaluate with precision the impact of their own policies and procedures on costs and quality of care for given beneficiary groups. This problem is exacerbated by the chronic instability of this rather young and entrepreneurial industry—a state of flux caused by companies constantly merging, being purchased, or purchasing other companies.

These issues must come to be explicitly addressed as part of the contract between the employer and the managed care company. Contacts themselves must reflect the longer-term view. Until each party demonstrates an ongoing commitment to effective communication and strategic thinking, as well as to continuous monitoring and periodic formal review of managed care performance objectives, the seriously damaging effects of "shopping around" by employers will continue, to the detriment of employer, managed care company, and beneficiary.

CONCLUSION

Managed care programs provide systematic approaches to controlling the delivery of previously uncontrolled behavioral health services. A principal consequence of managed systems is restrictions on the degree of autonomy previously exercised by service providers in independent practice—a group for whom autonomy is a primary professional value (Tryon, 1983). No matter what the strengths of managed systems, then, their arrival was bound to be met with acrimony on the part of providers.

What have been the contributions of managed care? Even among those people who develop and operate managed care companies there is a difference of opinion about issues such as the extent to which managed care has thus far affected the quality of services, to what extent these companies are driven by cost versus clinical concerns, and the distribution of quality across the managed care companies themselves. Nonetheless, one indisputable contribution of the industry has been its substantial, albeit indirect, role in diagnosing the problems of traditional health services delivery. Managed care programs have helped illuminate the problems endemic in the fee-for-service approach to financing.

While providers, payers, and managed care companies all seem to have different, and strongly held, opinions about the nature of problems of the fee-for-service system and their source, it is very clear that all stakeholders bear a measure of responsibility for the crisis in behavioral health services which provided the impetus for managed approaches. As

Troy (1994) states, each stakeholder group has contributed differentially to the malaise. For example:

- The professional education community has consistently failed to prepare students for the world of practice.
- The professional associations have made few serious attempts at accountability through promulgation of effective standards for education, training, and practice; they have vigorously opposed, rather than attempted to shape, the development of managed care; and they have maintained steadfast—and largely unexamined—support for generic psychotherapy as an effective health services intervention.
- The provider communities have been reluctant to embrace the principles of accountability; have maintained a resolute commitment to generic psychotherapy as a cure-all; and have largely abandoned organized care settings and the public sector care ethic.
- Managed care companies, at least in their earlier days, gave insufficient commitment to controlling the quality and acceptability of the case management process; were insufficiently discriminating in provider selection and monitoring; provided inadequate on-the-job training and professional development for network practitioners and case managers; and, in some cases, focused more on price competition than competition based on quality of services.
- Consumers, no doubt encouraged by service providers, have had unrealistic expectations about what behavioral health services can do for them, and at what price.
- Governments, particularly within the past decade, have neglected the health and social services infrastructure, science and education, and the health needs of under served groups.

Looking to the Future

A climate of change pervades health services in the U.S. Whether the prevailing approach to health services delivery and financing within the next decade will be bona fide "managed competition" or a mix of hybrid models and price controls, there is no doubt that management principles as discussed in this book will be central. Irrespective of the particular structures which emerge, an inevitable consequence of reform will be alliance-building among key stakeholder groups. Indeed, the capacity of the managed care industry to compete on quality rather than on price alone will ensure an increasing rapprochement between the managed care companies and various provider groups. And, whether or not these stakeholders find it palatable, the exemplar for such a union still remains the best of the staff or group model HMOs. No other arrangement has yet managed to create a system in which so many of the antecedents of quality of care are simultaneously present. Yet, acceptability of these systems (in the form of expressed satisfaction) to system providers and consumers alike has not tended to be the strong suit of the HMO. The climate of reform may yet see certain managed care companies come increasingly to resemble hybrid HMO systems. The pressure to improve the control of variation—a cornerstone of quality improvement—will be the force driving such a development.

As we have seen, the managed behavioral health care industry would do well not to rely too heavily upon the professional education and training community for a continuous supply of competent new providers. The industry itself will undoubtedly seek to establish partnerships with certain enterprising and innovative training programs.

At their best such partnerships carry clear advantages for both parties. The training program acquires the means (field training, professional role models, viable research options) for it truly to deliver a finished product—a graduate clinical professional with knowledge, skills, and attitudes/values appropriate to the changing world of managed health care and to the consumers supported by such a world. In turn, the managed care company receives for its efforts academic consultants to contribute to system evaluation, quality assessment, and management; a "quality-assured" source of providers; and the opportunity to influence directly the professional curricula, together with the chance for certain system providers to occupy academic roles within the training programs as valued clinical associate faculty.

Whatever the new structural arrangements the industry has yet to witness, and whatever the kind of alliances which develop among representatives of stakeholder communities, the signal development will be—indeed, will have to be—a vast change in the professional competency armamentarium of providers. Within the set of competencies, it will be changes in the attitudes/values of providers that will be paramount. Of particular interest will be the new ways providers will come to construe their professional roles, roles largely influenced by the changing structure of the context in which they will be embedded. Fundamental to this changing professional persona will be a value shift from the rather simple, direct rewards of independent practice, including its traditional autonomy, to the more complex, subtle and altruistic rewards of working within true systems—roles where accountability to consumers and sanctioners is manifest and guaranteed by a central place for quality management. Providers will become technical and systems consultants and applied researchers, in addition to their direct care involvement.

Finally, it might be expected that the very nature of the field of behavioral health will change. Currently a pragmatic amalgam of mental health and chemical dependency services, behavioral health has yet to find an identity beyond this *ad hoc* arrangement. It will take time, but it will surely encompass a multifaceted set of services embracing health psychology and behavioral medicine, prevention and health promotion, within a public health ethic. It will have its own rigorous empirical science base, research and practice norms, as well as a cadre of skilled and disciplined professional practitioners constructing a unique tradition of training and professional development.

Typically, professions evolve and financing systems evolve to suit them. It is both exciting and sobering to realize that it appears to be the integrated financing and service systems unique to managed care that are driving the development of a profession, and its identity. This is a profound change and it is inexorable. In an important way, things will never again be the same for the providers of mental health and chemical dependency services.

REFERENCES

Follette, W. & Cummings, N. (1967). Psychiatric services and medical utilization in a prepaid health plan setting. *Medical Care, 5,* 25–35.

Milstein, A., Henderson, M., Berlant, J., & Anderson, D. (1994). Evaluating psychiatric and substance abuse case management organizations. In S. Shueman, W. Troy, & S. Mayhugh (Eds.), *Managed Behavioral Health Care: An Industry Perspective.* Springfield, Illinois: Charles C Thomas, 222–240.

Rodriguez, A. (1989). Evolutions in utilization and quality management. *General Hospital Psychiatry, 11,* 256–263.

Troy, W.G. (1994). Developing and improving professional competencies. In S. Shueman, W. Troy, & S. Mayhugh (Eds.), *Managed Behavioral Health Care: An Industry Perspective.* Springfield, Illinois: Charles C Thomas, 168–188.

Tryon, G.S. (1983). Pleasures and displeasures of full-time private practice. *The Clinical Psychologist, 36*(4), 45–48.

AUTHOR INDEX

A

Adler, D.A., 10, 38
Adler, T., 101, 111
Anderson, Donald F., v, xx, 192, 222, 247, 256
Anderson, G.M., 161, 163
Appelbaum, P.S., 187
Applebaum, 178
Asher, J., 12, 27, 33, 35, 43
Attkisson, C.C., 213, 219
Auerbach, A., 212, 219
Austad, C.S., 70, 71, 75, 178, 187
Ausubel, David, 173

B

Bassuck, E., 238, 240
Batini, C., 197, 204
Battle, C., 212, 213, 219
Beck, Aaron T., 152, 163, 212, 219
Belar, C.D., 175, 176, 178, 187
Bennett, M.J., 99, 104, 111
Bent, R.J., 16, 27, 161, 163, 173, 187
Bent, Russell L., xvii
Bergin, A., 75
Berlant, Jeffrey L., v, xx, 10, 192, 222, 247, 256
Berman, W.H., 68, 75, 111
Berwick, D.M., 132, 145, 146, 147, 163
Binder, J., 68, 75
Biskin, B.H., 157, 163
Blackwell, B., 172, 175, 178, 187
Boaz, J.T., 176, 178, 187
Boland, Peter, iii, v, xii, xix
Bradley, W.J., 207, 219
Bricklin, P.M., 64
Brook, Robert H., xvii, 214, 219
Broskowski, A., 67, 74, 75
Buie, J., 103, 107, 111
Bulatao, Elizabeth Q., v, xix, 95, 97, 111

Bush, George, 98

C

Callan, J.E., 163, 187
Campbell, D.T., 234, 240
Carlisle, D.M., 108, 111
Carter, Jimmy, 106, 110
Carveth, B.W., 26, 27
Ceri, S., 197, 204
Cheifetz, D.I., 104, 108, 111
Christianson, J.D., 105, 112
Claiborn, W.L., 157, 163
Clements, C.B., 178, 187
Collins, M.F., 97, 99, 112
Cook, T., 114, 125
Crits-Christoph, P., 212, 219
Cuerdon, T., 105, 112
Cummings, Nicholas A., v, xvii, xx, 70, 72, 75, 105, 111, 114, 125, 191, 205, 206, 207, 217, 219, 220, 245

D

Darling, H., 23, 28
Davies-Avery, A., 214, 219
DeLeon, Patrick H., v, xix, 22, 28, 68, 75, 95, 97, 106, 111, 112
Deming, W.E., 132, 145, 147
Divine, E., 114, 125
Domnick-Pierre, K., 161, 163
Donabedian, Avedis, xvii, 132, 136, 145, 147, 149, 161, 163
Dörken, Herbert, v, xx, 96, 113, 117, 126, 217, 220
Dowling, W.L., 100, 112
Doyle, R., 198, 204

257

SUBJECT INDEX

A

Accountability, public (*see* Public accountability)

Administrative services only plan, 20

Advanced PsychSystems (APS), origin of, 42

American Psychiatric Association, work with DoD/CHAMPUS officials, 33–34

American Psychological Association, work with DoD/CHAMPUS officials, 33–34

Automated management information system, 193–203
  advantages of, 193
  conclusion, 202
  criteria to discontinue analysis, 201
  entities and associated attributes in, table, 202
  functions of automation, 196–200
  reasons for using, 193–195
  structure of entity database, 201–202
  support case management activities of, 195–196

B

Behavioral health care providers (*see also* Managed behavioral health care)
  adaptation to managed health care, ix (*see also* Managed health care)
    issues regarding, ix–x
  integration with primary medical care, x–xi
  lack benefits of graduate training programs, 185
  lack accountability in 1970s, 5
  need redefine role and value of, xi
  problems of, 9
  services defined, 9

Behavioral health case review, 76–91

case management company, 78–91 (*see also* Case management)
  effect case management on cost, 77–78
  goals of case management, 76–77
  role manager of services, 78–79
  role of service provider, 78–79

C

Case management, 78–91
  direct intervention with patient, example, 90–91
  identification cases requiring, 84–87
    case example, 84–87
    criteria for, table, 85
  model of, 79–84
    case example, 81–84
    range of utilization management activities, 80
  professional status issues, 89–90
    example, 89
  responsibilities of, 78, 79
  rewards from work, 90–91
  role of case manager, 87–89
  utilization review (*see* Utilization review)

CHAMPUS (Civilian Health and Medical Program of the Uniformed Services)
  and managed care, 101–104
  cost overruns of, 32–33
  development peer review program, 36–37 (*see also* Peer review program)
  efforts to managed care approach, 102–103
  frequency of case review, 123
  government as purchaser, 101–104
  growth of, 103
  increasing costs of, 102
  limitations on mental health benefits, 36
  origin of practice guidelines, 157–158
  pioneering role of, 29–37

261

END